D0077260

MILADY'S STANDARD
COSMETOLOGY
THEORY
WORKBOOK

MILADY'S STANDARD
COSMETOLOGY
THEORY
WORKBOOK

To be used with
MILADY'S STANDARD COSMETOLOGY

Compiled by
Catherine Frangie

THOMSON
™
DELMAR LEARNING

AUSTRALIA   CANADA   MEXICO   SINGAPORE   SPAIN   UNITED KINGDOM   UNITED STATES

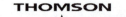

THOMSON
DELMAR LEARNING

Milady's Standard Cosmetology Theory Workbook
Compiled by Catherine Frangie

COPYRIGHT © 2004 by Milady, an imprint of Delmar, a division of Thomson Learning, Inc. Thomson Learning™ is a trademark used herein under license

Printed in the United States of America
  4 5 6 7 8 9 10 XXX 06 05 04

For more information contact Milady,
Executive Woods, 5 Maxwell Drive
Clifton Park, New York 12065-2919

Or find us on the World Wide Web at http://www.milady.com

All rights reserved. No part of this work covered by the copyright hereon may be reproduced or used in any form or by any means—graphic, electronic, or mechanical, including photocopying, recording, taping, Web distribution or information storage and retrieval systems—without written permission of the publisher.

For permission to use material from this text or product, contact us by
Tel   (800) 730-2214
Fax   (800) 730-2215
www.thomsonrights.com

Library of Congress Catalog Card Number: 2002074216
ISBN 1-56253-890-X

NOTICE TO THE READER

Publisher does not warrant or guarantee any of the products described herein or perform any independent analysis in connection with any of the product information contained herein. Publisher does not assume, and expressly disclaims, any obligation to obtain and include information other than that provided to it by the manufacturer.

The reader is expressly warned to consider and adopt all safety precautions that might be indicated by the activities herein and to avoid all potential hazards. By following the instructions contained herein, the reader willingly assumes all risks in connection with such instructions.

The Publisher makes no representation or warranties of any kind, including but not limited to, the warranties of fitness for particular purpose or merchantability, nor are any such representations implied with respect to the material set forth herein, and the publisher takes no responsibility with respect to such material. The publisher shall not be liable for any special, consequential, or exemplary damages resulting, in whole or part, from the readers' use of, or reliance upon, this material.

CONTENTS

D0077262

How to Use This Workbook

Milady's Standard Cosmetology Theory Workbook has been written to meet the needs, interests, and abilities of students receiving training in cosmetology.

This workbook should be used together with *Milady's Standard Cosmetology* and *Milady's Standard Cosmetology Practical Workbook*. This book directly follows the theoretical information found in the student textbook. Pages to be read and studied are listed at the beginning of each chapter. The practical information can be found in *Milady's Standard Cosmetology Practical Workbook*.

Students are to answer each item in this workbook with a pencil after consulting their textbook for correct information. Items can be corrected and/or rated during class or individual discussions, or on an independent study basis.

Various tests are included to emphasize essential facts found in the textbook and to measure the student's progress.

COSMETOLOGY:
THE HISTORY AND OPPORTUNITIES

Date: _____

Rating:_____

Text Pages: 3-19

POINT TO PONDER

"Education today, more than ever before, must see clearly the dual objective: Educating for living and educating for making a living." - James Mason Woods

REACHING YOUR GOALS

1. What is the single most important element of your quest for success?

   _____

2. To get the greatest benefits from your education, what commitments must you make?

   a) _____

   b) _____

   c) _____

   d) _____

   e) _____

   f) _____

   g) _____

   h) _____

   i) _____

3. What are the emotional requirements of making a lifelong career out of cosmetology?

   _____

   _____

EARLY HISTORY

4. The term "cosmetology" is derived from the Greek word kosmetikos. What is its meaning?

   _____

5. The term "barber" is derived from the Latin word barba. What is its meaning?

   _____

6. How did the ancient Egyptians first use cosmetics?

   _____

7. The ancient Egyptians used _____, a natural dye extracted from the leaves of an ornamental shrub, to impart a reddish tint to the hair.

8. What mixture did Egyptian and Roman women use to create a temporary wave in their hair?

   _____

   _____

9. When was the first evidence of nail care recorded in history and where was it recorded?

   _____

10. In ancient Egypt the color of a person's nails was a sign of rank. What color did kings and queens

    wear? _____ What color did people of lower status wear? _____

11. When did hairstyling become a highly developed art?

    _____ a) 250 B.C.
    _____ b) 500 B.C.
    _____ c) 750 B.C.
    _____ d) 1000 B.C.

12. In Rome around 300 B.C. women used hair color to indicate their class in society. Match the correct shade with its corresponding class.

    _____ 1. noblewomen   A. black
    _____ 2. middle-class women   B. red
    _____ 3. poor women   C. blond

13. Why were barbers enlisted to assist monks and priests during surgery?

_____

_____

14. Who performed dentistry in medieval times? What were they called?

_____

15. When did hairstyling begin to emerge as an independent profession and why?

_____

_____

_____

16. _____ developed a technique using irons for waving and curling the hair. This practice developed into the art of thermal waving, which is still known today as _____.

17. When was the hot-blast hairdryer invented and by whom?

_____

THE TWENTIETH CENTURY

18. Before the twentieth century, hairstyling and makeup were used to indicate:

a) _____

b) _____

c) _____

d) _____

e) _____

19. How did hairstyling change after the twentieth century?

_____

_____

20. _____ was a pioneer of the modern black hair-care and cosmetics industry.

21. _____ invented a heavily wired machine that supplied electrical current to metal rods around which hair strands were wrapped. These heavy units were heated during the waving process. This process became the first _____.

22. Winding long hair from the scalp to the ends is a wrapping technique called _____. Winding short hair from the ends toward the scalp is called _____.

23. The first machine-less permanent wave was invented in _____ by _____ and _____, two chemists who pioneered a method that used external heat generated by chemical reaction to curl hair.

24. What is a cold wave?

_____

25. The terms _____ and _____ have become almost synonymous.

CAREER OPPORTUNITIES

26. Match each of the following job descriptions with the correct title:

_____ 1.	performs all the services offered in the salon	A. platform artist
_____ 2.	creates color formulations and techniques	B. cosmetic chemist
_____ 3.	changes the hair's texture	C. salon manager
_____ 4.	creates hairstyles by adding or replacing hair	D. makeup artist
_____ 5.	handles and sells merchandise	E. nail technician/manicurist
_____ 6.	treats the look and health of the skin	F. educator
_____ 7.	applies cosmetics to enhance appearance	G. design team member
_____ 8.	offers manicure, pedicures and extensions	H. retail specialist
_____ 9.	focuses on overall appearance and health	I. salon stylist
_____ 10.	oversees all aspects of salon service and staff	J. hair color specialist
_____ 11.	oversees all aspects of business operations	K. skin care specialist/esthetician
_____ 12.	sells and demonstrates products to professionals	L. texture service specialist
_____ 13.	creates and formulates new products	M. day spa stylist or technician
_____ 14.	styles hair and makeup for photography	N. wig or extensions specialist
_____ 15.	creates company/product image through hair artistry	O. competition champion
_____ 16.	works with a team to create styles for presentation	P. salon owner
_____ 17.	educator who performs techniques at major hair events	Q. product educator
_____ 18.	trains and hones techniques for competition	R. styles director/artistic director
_____ 19.	one who trains others	S. session hairstylist

DISCUSSION QUESTIONS

29. Why have you chosen a career in cosmetology?

_____

_____

2

LIFE SKILLS

Date: _____

Rating: _____

Text Pages: 21-43

POINT TO PONDER:

"What I am thinking and doing day by day is resistlessly shaping my future—a future in which there is no expiation except through my own better conduct. No one can live my life for me; if I am wise I shall begin today to build my own truer and better world from within."—H.W. Dresser

1. What are "life skills?"

   _____

   _____

2. Below is a list of different life skills. Put a check mark next to the skills you feel you are well on your way to mastering, and put a circle next to the ones you need to improve.

   _____ being genuinely caring and helpful to other people

   _____ successfully adapting to different situations

   _____ sticking to a goal and seeing a job to completion

   _____ developing common sense

   _____ making good friends and feeling good about yourself

   _____ maintaining a cooperative attitude in all situations

   _____ defining "courage" for yourself and living courageously within your definition

   _____ approaching all your work and personal matters with a strong sense of responsibility

   _____ learning techniques that will help you become more organized

   _____ having a sense of humor to bring you through difficult situations

   _____ acquiring that great virtue known as "patience"

   _____ consistently making an effort in any projects you undertake and always striving for excellence

   _____ dedicating yourself to becoming an honest and trustworthy individual.

THE PSYCHOLOGY OF SUCCESS

3. A common characteristic shared by most successful people is that they _____ .

4. How is self-esteem related to success?

   _____

   _____

5. People who talk about themselves or others at work promote an excellent environment for teamwork.

   _____ True

   _____ False

6. Compartmentalization is the ability to store things away in the different compartments of the mind.

   _____ True

   _____ False

7. Circle the correct answer: Successful people do/do not run themselves ragged, and they

   do/do not eat, sleep, and drink business. They do/do not take time to meet their human needs,

   like spending time with family and friends, exercising, and eating a good, nutritious diet. They

   do/do not know that success means having a clear head, a fit body, and the ability to refuel

   and recharge.

8. List three ways to show respect for others:

   a) _____

   b) _____

   c) _____

   _____

9. Unscramble these terms and then match them with their definition below.

   naotiostcrinpra   mfepnictsioer   eagm apln

   _____   To put off until tomorrow what you can do today.

   _____   The compulsion to do things perfectly all of the time.

   _____   The conscious act of planning your life rather than just

                                letting things happen.

MOTIVATION AND SELF-MANAGEMENT

10. _____ is the ignition for success. _____ is the fuel that will keep you

going on the long ride to your destination.

11. What is the difference between motivation and self-management?

_____

_____

12. Where does motivation come from?

_____

_____

13. When you find yourself asking "Why do I need to know this? How is this material going to help me in my career?" What should you remember?

_____

_____

_____

14. List some physical needs.

_____

15. Name some emotional needs.

_____

16. Name some social needs.

_____

17. Name a mental need:

_____

18. Name a spiritual need.

_____

19. Define creativity. Where does it come from?

_____

_____

_____

20. Name four ways you can enhance the skill of creativity in your life.

    a) _____   c) _____

    b) _____   d) _____

MANAGING YOUR CAREER

21. What is a mission statement, and how is it useful to you personally?

_____

_____

GOAL SETTING

22. Goal-setting helps you decide what you want out of your life.

    _____ True

    _____ False

23. An example of a short-term goal is to successfully open and manage your own salon.

    _____ True

    _____ False

24. An example of a long-term goal is to graduate from beauty school.

    _____ True

    _____ False

25. In order to achieve my goals I will need to (check all that apply):

_____ learn additional, specific skills

_____ gather more information

_____ ask others for help

_____ seek out a mentor or a coach to enhance my learning

_____ determine the best method or approach to accomplishing my goals

_____ become open to finding better ways of putting my plan into practice

TIME MANAGEMENT

26. Put a check mark next to each of the following time management techniques that you would like to include or further develop in your life:

_____ prioritizing tasks

_____ designing my own time management system

_____ reducing stress

_____ not taking on more than I can handle

_____ learning problem-solving techniques that save time by uncovering solutions

_____ giving myself free time to regroup

_____ take notes of my thoughts and ideas

_____ make schedules for my regular commitments

_____ reward myself for good work

_____ make physical activity a regular part of my life

_____ use to-do lists to prioritize tasks and activities

_____ make time management a habit

STUDY SKILLS

27. If you find it difficult to study for long periods of time, what might you try instead?

_____

_____

28. What can you do if you find your mind wanders in class?

_____

_____

29. What is a study buddy?

_____

_____

30. _____ do best when they can ask "Why?" They learn by watching, listening, and

    sharing ideas.

31. _____ ask "What?" They learn best by reading as well as hearing new ideas

    and then mulling over the information in their minds.

32. When _____ sit down to study, they get more out of the information when they

    can connect what they are studying to real-life situations.

33. _____ ask "What if...?" They like to learn through trial and error.

ETHICS

34. Ethics are the principles of _____ , _____ ,

    and _____ , expressed through _____ , _____ ,

    and _____ .

35. Professionals practice the following qualities: _____ , _____ , _____

    and _____ .

PERSONALITY DEVELOPMENT AND ATTITUDE

36. Your _____ defines who you are. It is the way you walk and talk; the way you hold your

    head, it is what distinguishes you from another person.

37. Your _____ can be defined as your outlook. It stems from what you believe, and it can be

    influenced by your parents, teachers, friends, and even books and movies.

38. What are the "ingredients" of a healthy, well-developed attitude?

    _____

    _____

HUMAN RELATIONS

39. It is always possible to get along with everyone.

_____   True
_____   False

40. A fundamental factor in human relations has to do with how _____ we are feeling. When we

feel _____ , we are _____ , _____ , and _____ , and we act in a

_____ and _____ manner.

41. What five things should you always keep in mind when dealing with others, especially in an emotional situation?

a) _____   d) _____

b) _____   e) _____

c) _____

DISCUSSION QUESTIONS

For each of these questions, answer honestly and share your answers with your class at the appropriate time for discussion.

42. How do you personally define success?

_____

43. Describe below how you visualize yourself in beauty school. How do you visualize yourself one year from now?

_____

44. List three things you know you are good at:

a. _____

b. _____

c. _____

45. List three things about which you'd like to be kinder to yourself.

    a. _____

    b. _____

    c. _____

46. List three new, positive behaviors you would like to practice.

    a. _____

    b. _____

    c. _____

47. Below, write a mission statement in one or two sentences that communicates who you are and what

    you want in your life between now and the time you graduate from school.

    _____

48. List three things you are working toward at this time in your life.

    a. _____

    b. _____

    c. _____

49. List three short-term goals:

    a. _____

    b. _____

    c. _____

50. List three long-term goals:

    a. _____

    b. _____

    c. _____

51. When it comes to studying, where do you have difficulty?

    _____

3
YOUR PROFESSIONAL IMAGE

Date: _____

Rating: _____

Text Pages: 45-65

POINT TO PONDER:

"A fresh mind keeps the body fresh. Take in the ideas of the day, drain off those of yesterday. As to the morrow, time enough to consider it when it becomes today."—Bulwer

1. Image is a combination of our _____ —how we look to the world—with

who we are deep inside, or _____.

2. Your professional image should convey to your clients that you are cool and hip.

   _____ True
   _____ False

3. What is a holistic image and how is it achieved?

   _____

   _____

BEAUTY AND WELLNESS

4. As a cosmetologist and a beauty and wellness consultant, you are also a _____ ,

   and as such, your first concern is to take care of _____ so that you can go on to take care

   of others.

5. How do you know if you are in good health?

   _____

   _____

6. To remain healthy, you must remain in balance. Which of the following is an example of making a balanced decision?

_____ a) eating poorly

_____ b) drinking excessively

_____ c) letting go of toxic emotions

_____ d) smoking

7. Unscramble these words and place them in the sentence below:

onpalrse   igeehny

_____ is the daily maintenance of cleanliness and healthfulness through certain

sanitary practices.

8. It is not necessary to do which of the following every day?

_____ a) bathe or shower

_____ b) wash your hands

_____ c) use underarm deodorant or antiperspirant

_____ d) visit the dentist

9. A very important element of your image as a professional cosmetologist is:

_____ a) a cell phone

_____ b) a designer outfit

_____ c) well-groomed hair

_____ d) a leather briefcase

10. What kind of attitude is projected by chipped nails, unkempt hair and sloppy grooming?

_____

11. Many salon owners and managers consider _____ , _____ ,

and _____ to be just as important for success as technical knowledge and skills.

12. One of the most important aspects of good personal grooming is the careful maintenance of your wardrobe.

    _____ True

    _____ False

13. In regards to your style, what will you want to determine about a salon when interviewing for possible employment?

    _____

    _____

14. Your hairstyle should always be funky and "cutting-edge" to show clients that you are trendy.

    _____ True

    _____ False

15. You should never color or perm your hair when you work in a salon.

    _____ True

    _____ False

16. What is the best approach to facial makeup a female cosmetologist can take?

    _____

    _____

HEALTHY MIND AND BODY

17. What is stress?

    _____

    _____

18. Which of the following techniques can be used to handle stress no matter what the situation?

    _____ a) 20 minutes of meditation

    _____ b) a yoga class

    _____ c) deep breathing

    _____ d) repeating positive affirmations aloud

19. It is essential to get enough _____ and _____ in order for your body to function

efficiently.

20. Why is good nutrition important?

_____

_____

21. List four basic guidelines for good nutrition.

a) _____

b) _____

c) _____

d) _____

22. Which of the following is considered a fat?

_____ a) apple

_____ b) butter

_____ c) bread

_____ d) salmon

23. Which of the following is considered a carbohydrate?

_____ a) apple

_____ b) butter

_____ c) bread

_____ d) salmon

24. Which of the following is considered a protein?

_____ a) apple

_____ b) butter

_____ c) bread

_____ d) salmon

25. Which of the following is considered a fruit or vegetable?

_____ a) apple

_____ b) butter

_____ c) bread

_____ d) salmon

26. An adequate amount of physical activity ensures the _____ of organs such

as the heart and lungs, strengthens _____, enhances immune function, and

improves_____.

27. List the three main types of activity:

a) _____

_____

b) _____

_____

c) _____

_____

YOUR PHYSICAL PRESENTATION

28. Physical presentation is made up of your:

_____ a) posture, walk, and movements.

_____ b) hair color, length and style.

_____ c) nail length, shape and design.

_____ d) skin texture, tone and elasticity.

29. Taking good care of your feet means that you must _____

_____.

30. Which of the following is the study of human characteristics for a specific work environment?

    _____ a) aeronautics

    _____ b) economics

    _____ c) ergonomics

    _____ d) philosophic

DISCUSSION QUESTIONS

Answer the following questions and be prepared to discuss them in class at the appropriate time.

31. What is your personal sense of style?

    _____

32. Describe below how you cope with stress.

    _____

33. List three ways in which you relax:

    a. _____

    b. _____

    c. _____

4

COMMUNICATING FOR SUCCESS

Date: _____

Rating:_____

Text Pages: 67-90

POINT TO PONDER:

"Wisdom is knowing when to speak your mind and when to mind your speech."—Evangel

COMMUNICATION BASICS

1. _____ is the best way of ensuring that you understand perfectly the

    needs, wants, and desires of the people around you.

2. Communication is the act or instance of _____, in the form of

    symbols, gestures, or behaviors, in order to express an idea or concept so that it is satisfactorily

    understood.

3. What are the three basic processes of communicating?

    a) _____

    b) _____

    c) _____

4. The first step in the communication process is to collect your_____

    —what you want others to understand.

5. Unscramble these words and use them to fill in the blanks in the sentence below:

    lattresan   lsbomsy

    The second step in communicating is to _____ those thoughts and feelings into

    _____ that can be easily understood by others.

6. Helping a client to clearly express his desires is called:

   _____ a) manipulation

   _____ b) capitulation

   _____ c) articulation

   _____ d) infatuation

   _____ d) infatuation

7. What types of symbols are used in everyday communication?

   _____

   _____

8. What does it mean to clarify the message and how do you do it?

   _____

   _____

9. To prove that you have heard and understand your client you should use a technique called

   _____, whereby you repeat in your own words what you believe your client

   just told you. This will determine whether the two of you are on the same page or not.

10. In addition to clarifying and reflecting, the next step in interpreting your client's message involves

    _____.

11. The final step in the interpretation process consists of reading all the clues and symbols the client is
    putting out.

    _____ True

    _____ False

THE CLIENT CONSULTATION

12. What is a client consultation?

    _____

    _____

13. How often should a client consultation be performed?

_____ a) never

_____ b) every visit

_____ c) every other visit

_____ d) only for hair color services

14. What tools should you prepare for use in the client consultation?

a) _____

b) _____

c) _____

15. The Total Look Concept involves _____

_____ .

16. How long should a nail consultation take?

_____

_____

17. How detailed should a skin care consultation be?

_____

18. The purpose of a consultation card is to _____

_____ .

19. The client consultation card should be updated:

_____ a) never

_____ b) every visit

_____ c) every other visit

_____ d) only for hair color services

20. The ideal setting for a consultation is _____

_____ .

21. When is the best time to look over the information the client has provided on the consultation card?

    _____

    _____

22. The best way to clarify what your clients are saying is to lecture them.

    _____ True
    _____ False

23. Throughout the _____ make notes and record any _____ or _____

    that you use, and include any _____ you follow or goals you are working

    toward so that you can remember them for future visits.

SPECIAL ISSUES IN COMMUNICATION

24. When meeting and greeting clients you should be: _____

25. To earn the trust and loyalty of a new client you must:_____

    _____

    _____

26. List ways in which tardy clients be handled so that you don't lose their business or ruin your day's schedule.

    a) _____

    b) _____

    c) _____

    d) _____

27. When a scheduling mix-up occurs you should:

    _____ Not admit that you or anyone in the salon made the mistake.

    _____ Argue with the client about who wrote the appointment down incorrectly.

    _____ Be polite and never argue the point of which one of you is correct.

    _____ Blame the salon's receptionist and call the manager.

28. If you master all your hairdressing skills perfectly, you will never have an unhappy client.

    _____ True
    _____ False

29. Which of the following are appropriate ways of dealing with unhappy clients? (check all that apply)

_____ find out just why the client is unhappy

_____ do not change what the client dislikes until their next visit

_____ change whatever the client does not like, even if it might damage her hair

_____ call on a more experienced stylist or your salon manager for help

IN-SALON COMMUNICATION

30. What is the value of building good relationships with your coworkers and managers?

_____

31. What are the most important things to remember as you interact and communicate with fellow staffers?

a) _____

b) _____

c) _____

d) _____

e) _____

f) _____

g) _____

32. What is your salon manager's most important job?

_____

_____

33. What things should you strive for when dealing with your manager?

a) _____

b) _____

c) _____

d) _____

e) _____

f) _____

34. What kinds of salons conduct frequent and thorough employee evaluations?

_____

35. An employee evaluation is done secretly and the employee never gets to see the evaluation form.

_____ True

_____ False

36. As the time draws near for the evaluation, what should you do?

_____ a) ask your manager to postpone the meeting

_____ b) fill out the form yourself

_____ c) apply for a new job in a different salon

_____ d) make a list of complaints you have about how the salon is managed

37. What kinds of things are discussed in an evaluation meeting?

a) _____

b) _____

c) _____

38. Why do many beauty professionals never take advantage of this crucial communication opportunity?

_____

39. When in a performance evaluation meeting it is best to:

_____ a) let your manager do all of the talking

_____ b) listen to your manager's feedback and ask for clarification when it's needed

_____ c) allow your manager to discuss other employees' performance

_____ d) share complaints about fellow staffers with your manager

40. At the end of the meeting, you should _____

_____.

5

INFECTION CONTROL: PRINCIPLES AND PRACTICE

Date: _____

Rating:_____

Text Pages: 93-127

POINT TO PONDER:

"One pound of learning requires ten pounds of common sense to apply it."—Persian Proverb

BACTERIA

1. Bacteria are one-celled _____ with both plant and animal characteristics. Also known

    as _____ or _____ , bacteria can exist almost anywhere: on the skin, in water, air,

    decayed matter, secretions of body openings, on clothing, and beneath the nails.

2. There are hundreds of different kinds of bacteria. They are classified into two main types, depending on
    whether they are beneficial or harmful.

    _____ True
    _____ False

3. Nonpathogenic organisms are helpful or harmless, not disease-producing, and they perform many

    useful functions, such as _____ and _____ .

    In the human body, nonpathogenic bacteria help _____ , protect against

    _____ , and stimulate _____ .

4. Pathogenic bacteria are harmful and, although in the minority, cause _____ when they invade

    plant or animal tissue. To this group belong the _____ , which require living matter for their

    growth.

5. Match each of the following bacteria with its unique shape:

_____	1. cocci	A.	string of beads
_____	2. staphylococci	B.	spheres
_____	3. streptococci	C.	corkscrews
_____	4. diplococci	D.	round
_____	5. bacilli	E.	grape-like clusters
_____	6. spirilla	F.	short rod shapes

6. Identify the forms of bacteria illustrated below.

1. _____ 2. _____ 3. _____

7. How do these bacteria move about?

cocci   _____

bacilli   _____

spirilla   _____

8. Unscramble these words and use them to complete the sentences below.

briateac   sopotparlm   atgeeetivv   cniatvie

_____ generally consist of an outer cell wall and internal _____. They

manufacture their own food from the surrounding environment, give off waste products, and grow and

reproduce. The life cycle of bacteria is made up of two distinct phases: the active or _____

stage, and the _____ or spore-forming stage.

9. During the active stage, bacteria:

_____ a) die

_____ b) grow

_____ c) change color

_____ d) dry out

10. This division of a bacteria cell is called _____. The cells that are formed are called

_____ .

11. Why do certain bacteria, such as the anthrax and tetanus bacilli, form spherical spores with tough outer coverings during their inactive stage?

_____

12. What occurs when body tissues are invaded by disease-causing or pathogenic bacteria?

_____

13. What is pus?

_____

_____

14. Which of the following is not a way that staphylococci are transmitted?

_____ a) touching a doorknob

_____ b) shaking hands

_____ c) brushing teeth

_____ d) using unclean implements

15. A _____ , such as a pimple or abscess, is one that is confined to a particular

part of the body and is indicated by a lesion containing pus. A _____ results when

the bloodstream carries the bacteria or virus and their toxins (poisons) to all parts of the body.

16. A communicable disease is also known as a _____ disease.

17. What are the chief sources of contagion?

a) _____   d) _____

b) _____   e) _____

c) _____   f) _____

VIRUSES

18. _____ are submicroscopic structures capable of infesting almost all plants and animals,

    including bacteria.

19. Viruses cause:

    a) _____   g) _____

    b) _____   h) _____

       _____   i) _____

    c) _____   j) _____

    d) _____   k) _____

    e) _____   l) _____

    f) _____

20. What's the difference between bacteria and viruses?

    _____

    _____

21. Hepatitis is a disease marked by _____ and caused by _____ .

22. Match the following form of hepatitis with its correct symptom:

    _____ 1. Hepatitis A   A. fatigue and stomach pain
    _____ 2. Hepatitis B   B. yellowing of the skin or eyes
    _____ 3. Hepatitis C   C. flu-like symptoms

HIV/AIDS

23. What does HIV stand for?

    _____

24. What does AIDS stand for?

    _____

25. How is the HIV virus transmitted?

   a) _____

   b) _____

   c) _____

26. Name some ways in which the HIV virus is not transmitted.

   _____

   _____

HOW PATHOGENS ENTER THE BODY

27. Pathogenic bacteria or viruses can enter the body through:

   a) _____

   b) _____

   c) _____

   d) _____

   e) _____

28. The body fights infection by means of:

   a) _____

   b) _____

   c) _____

   d) _____

29. Disease-causing bacteria or viruses that are carried through body in the blood or body fluids, such as

   hepatitis and HIV, are called_____ pathogens.

PARASITES

30. _____ are vegetable or animal organisms that live in or on another _____ organism

    and draw their _____ from that organism or _____ .

31. Vegetable _____ parasites or _____ , which include molds, mildews, and

    yeasts, can produce_____ diseases such as _____ and _____ .

32. Nail fungus can be contracted through implements that have not been _____ properly or

    by _____ trapped under nail enhancements. Nail fungus is _____ and

    usually localized but can be spread to other nails and from client to client if implements are not

    disinfected before and after each client.

33. A skin disease caused by an infestation of head lice is called _____ .

    _____ , another contagious skin disease, is caused by the itch mite, which burrows under

    the skin.

34. _____ diseases and conditions caused by parasites should_____ be treated in a

    cosmetology school or salon. Clients should be referred to a _____ .

IMMUNITY

35. Match each of the following terms with its correct definition.

    _____ 1. immunity   A. both an inherited and developed ability to destroy bacteria
    _____ 2. natural immunity   B. ability to overcome disease through inoculation
    _____ 3. acquired immunity   C. the body's ability to destroy bacteria

6

ANATOMY AND PHYSIOLOGY

Date: _____

Rating:_____

Text Pages: 129-165

POINT TO PONDER:

"Whoever acquires knowledge but does not practice it is as one who ploughs but does not sow."
—Saadi

1. _____ is the study of the structures of the human body that can be seen with the naked eye;

   it is the science of the structure of organisms or of their parts.

2. _____ is the study of the functions and activities performed by the body structures.

3. _____ is the study of the minute structures of organic tissues.

CELLS

4. What is a cell?

   _____

5. As a basic functional unit, the cell is responsible for carrying on all _____.

6. There are _____ of cells in the human body, and they vary widely in size, shape, and purpose.

   a) hundreds

   b) thousands

   c) millions

   d) trillions

7. Protoplasm is a colorless jellylike substance in which food elements such as _____ , _____ ,

   _____ , _____ , and _____ are present.

8. Unscramble these words and use them to fill in the blanks:

   ucsnelu   tosplacym   lelc emmarnbe

   a) The_____ is the dense, active protoplasm found in the center of the cell; it plays an

   important part in cell reproduction and metabolism.

   b) The_____ is all the protoplasm of a cell except that which is in the nucleus; the watery

   fluid that contains food material necessary for growth, reproduction, and self-repair of the cell.

   c) The_____ is the cell wall, a delicate protoplasmic material that encloses a living plant

   or animal cell and permits soluble substances to enter and leave the cell.

9. Identify the parts of the cell illustrated at right.

   a) _____

   b) _____

   c) _____

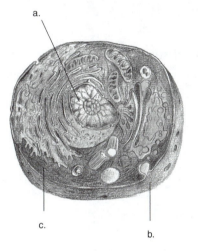

10. Cells have the ability to _____, thus providing new cells for the growth and replacement of

    worn or injured ones. Most cells reproduce by dividing into two identical cells called _____.

    This reproduction process is known as _____.

11. Metabolism is _____

    _____ .

12. Metabolism has two phases:

    a) _____

    b) _____

TISSUES

13. A tissue is a:

_____ a)   collection of similar cells that perform a particular function
_____ b)   single cell that destroys odor
_____ c)   protoplasm that nourishes cells
_____ d)   cell membrane

14. Match the correct tissue with its function:

_____ 1. Connective tissue   A. carries messages to and from the brain
_____ 2. Epithelial tissue   B. carries food, waste products, and hormones
                                          through the body
_____ 3. Liquid tissue   C. protective covering on body surfaces
_____ 4. Muscular tissue   D. supports, protects, and binds together
                                          other tissues
_____ 5. Nerve tissue   E. contracts and moves the various parts of the body

ORGANS

15. List the major organs of the body:

a) _____   e) _____

b) _____   f) _____

c) _____   g) _____

d) _____   h) _____

BODY SYSTEMS

16. Systems are groups of bodily _____ acting together to perform one or more functions.

17. Which of the following are systems?

_____ a)   stomach

_____ b)   arms

_____ c)   legs

_____ d)   endocrine

THE SKELETAL SYSTEM

18. The _____ is the physical foundation of the body.

19. The body is composed of _____ bones that vary in size and shape and are connected by movable and immovable joints.

    a) 87
    b) 124
    c) 206
    d) 292

20. The science of the anatomy, structure, and function of the bones is called _____ .

21. _____ is the hardest tissue in the body. It is composed of connective tissue consisting of about one-third animal matter, such as cells and blood, and two-thirds mineral matter, mainly calcium carbonate and calcium phosphate.

22. The primary functions of the skeletal system are to:

    a) _____

    b) _____

    c) _____

    d) _____

    e) _____

23. A pivot is the connection between two or more bones of the skeleton.

    _____ True

    _____ False

24. There are five main types of joints.

    _____ True

    _____ False

25. _____ joints are found in the elbows, knees, and hips; and _____ joints are found in the pelvis or skull.

26. The _____ is the skeleton of the head and is divided into two parts. These parts are the _____ an oval, bony case that protects the brain; and the _____ , which is made up of _____ bones.

27. There are _____ bones in the cranium:

    a) 3

    b) 6

    c) 8

    d) 10

28. Identify the bones of the cranium, face, and neck illustrated below.

    1. _____

    2. _____

    3. _____

    4. _____

    5. _____

    6. _____

    7. _____

    8. _____

    9. _____

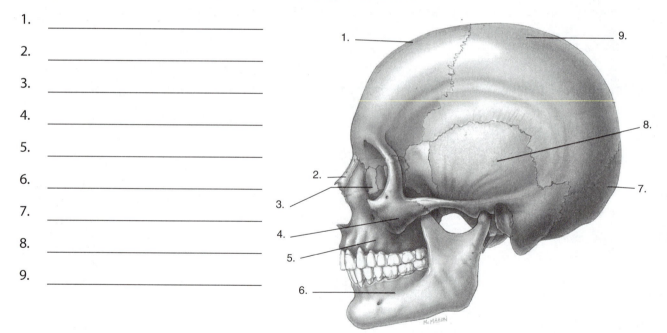

29. Match each of the following bones to its location.

    _____ 1. occipital bone   A. forehead
    _____ 2. parietal bones   B. sides of the head in the ear region
    _____ 3. frontal bone   C. back of the skull above the nape of the neck
    _____ 4. temporal bones   D. sides and crown (top) of the cranium

30. Where is each of these bones found?

nasal bones _____

lacrimal bones _____

zygomatic bones _____

maxillae _____

mandible _____

31. The main bones of the neck are: _____ .

32. The hyoid bone is also called the _____ .

a) nose

b) jaw

c) Adam's apple

d) eye socket

33. Match each of these bones with their location.

_____ 1. thorax   A. collarbone
_____ 2. ribs   B. chest
_____ 3. scapula   C. wall of the thorax
_____ 4. sternum   D. shoulder
_____ 5. clavicle   E. front of the ribs

34. Identify the bones of the neck, shoulder, and back as illustrated below.

1. _____

2. _____

3. _____

4. _____

5. _____

6. _____

7. _____

8. _____

35. The humerus is the _____ .

36. The ulna is the _____

_____ .

37. The radius is_____ .

38. The carpus is the _____ .

39. The metacarpus is made up the _____ .

40. The phalanges are _____ .

41. Identify the bones of the arm and hand illustrated below.

1. _____

2. _____

3. _____

4. _____

5. _____

1. _____

2. _____

3. _____

4. _____

5. _____

THE MUSCULAR SYSTEM

42. The muscular system is the body system that _____ , _____ , and _____

the skeleton tissue.

43. The human body has over _____ muscles, which are responsible for approximately 40% of the

    body's weight.

    a) 200

    b) 400

    c) 600

    d) 800

44. Muscles are fibrous tissues that have the ability to:

    _____ a)   create and destroy germs

    _____ b)   become warm and cold

    _____ c)   stretch and contract

    _____ d)   multiply and divide

45. The three types of muscular tissue are:

    a) _____

    b) _____

    c) _____

46. Striated muscles assist in maintaining the body's _____ and protect some _____ .

47. Nonstriated muscles are found in the _____ of the body, such as the _____
    or _____ .

48. Cardiac muscle is the _____ muscle that is found only in the heart. This type of muscle is not
    found in any other part of the body.

49. The origin of the muscle is_____
    _____ .

50. The insertion is _____ .

51. The belly is _____ .

52. In massage pressure is usually directed from the:

_____ a)　origin to the insertion

_____ b)　muscle to the bone

_____ c)　insertion to the origin

_____ d)　bone to the muscle

53. What are the ways that muscular tissue can be stimulated?

a) _____   e) _____

b) _____   f) _____

c) _____   g) _____

d) _____

54. The _____ is the broad muscle that covers the top of the skull. It consists of two parts, the

_____ and _____ .

55. What is the function of the occipitalis?

_____

56. What is the function of the frontalis?

_____

57. What is the function of the aponeurosis?

_____

58. Name the three muscles of the ear and their functions.

a) _____

b) _____

c) _____

59. What are the names of the muscles that coordinate in opening and closing the mouth and are sometimes referred to as chewing muscles?

_____

60. The _____ is a broad muscle extending from the chest and shoulder muscles

    to the side of the chin and is responsible for depressing the lower jaw and lip.

61. The _____ is a muscle of the neck that lowers and rotates the head.

62. Identify the muscles of the head and neck illustrated below.

   1. _____

   2. _____

   3. _____

   4. _____

   5. _____

   6. _____

   7. _____

   8. _____

   9. _____

   10. _____

   11. _____

   12. _____

   13. _____

   14. _____

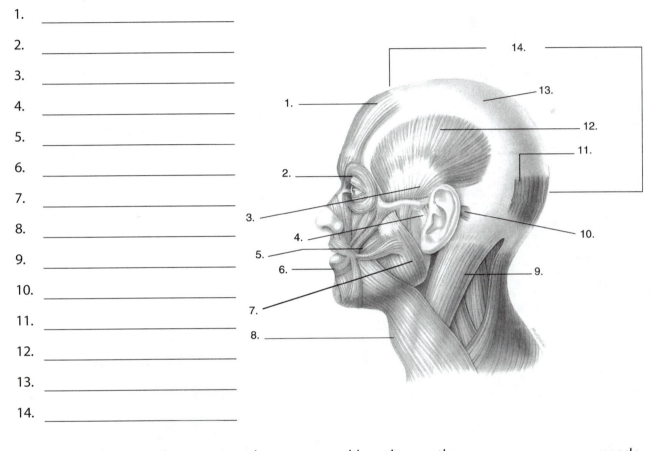

63. If you wanted to raise or lower your eyebrows you would need to use the _____ muscle.

    If you wanted to close your eyes you would need to use the _____ muscle.

64. The _____ muscle covers the bridge of the nose, lowers the eyebrows, and causes wrinkles

    across the bridge of the nose.

65. Match the following muscles of the mouth with their function:

_____ 1. buccinator

_____ 2. depressor labii inferioris

_____ 3. levator anguli oris

_____ 4. levator labii superioris

_____ 5. mentalis

_____ 6. orbicularis oris

_____ 7. risorius

_____ 8. triangularis

_____ 9. zygomaticus

A. elevates the lower lip and raises and wrinkles the skin of the chin

B. draws the corner of the mouth out and back

C. compresses the cheeks and expels air between the lips

D. compresses, contracts, puckers, and wrinkles the lips

E. depresses the lower lip and draws it to one side

F. raises the angle of the mouth and draws it inward

G. elevates the lip

H. elevates the upper lip and dilates the nostrils

I. pulls down the corner of the mouth

66. Identify the muscles of the head and neck as illustrated below.

1. _____

2. _____

3. _____

4. _____

5. _____

6. _____

7. _____

8. _____

9. _____

10. _____

11. _____

12. _____

13. _____

14. _____

15. _____

16. _____

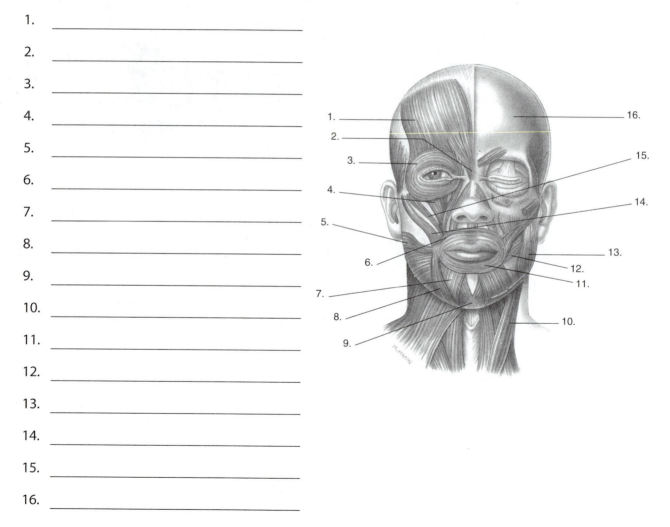

67. Name the four muscles that attach the arms to the body and the function of each:

    a) _____

    b) _____

    c) _____

    d) _____

68. Where is the biceps and what does it do?

    _____

    _____

69. Where is your deltoid muscle and what does it do?

    _____

    _____

70. Where are your triceps and what do they do?

    _____

71. Unscramble these words and use them to fill in the blanks below:

    trnaoorp   exfrslo   atpinsuor   eornsstex

    a) The_____ are the muscles that straighten the wrist, hand, and fingers to form a straight line.

    b) The_____ are the muscles of the wrist, involved in flexing the wrist.

    c) The_____ is the muscle that turns the hand inward so that the palm faces downward.

    d) The_____ is the muscle of the forearm that rotates the radius outward and the palm

    upward.

72. Identify the muscles of the shoulders, arms, and hands as illustrated below.

1. _____

2. _____

3. _____

4. _____

5. _____

Anterior or palm

73. To separate your fingers, you use the _____ muscles. To draw your fingers together you use

the _____ muscles. To move your thumb toward your fingers you use the _____

muscles.

THE NERVOUS SYSTEM

74. The three main subdivisions of the nervous system and their functions are:

a) _____

_____

b) _____

_____

c) _____

_____

75. Which of the following is not a component of a neuron?

_____ a) nucleus

_____ b) amoeba

_____ c) dendrites

_____ d) axon

76. Identify the parts of a neuron as illustrated below.

1. _____

2. _____

3. _____

4. _____

77. There are _____ types of nerves: _____ , which carry impulses or messages from the

sense organs to the brain; _____ , which carry impulses from the brain to the muscles;

and _____ , which contain both sensory and motor fibers and have the ability to send

and receive messages.

78. List the branches of the fifth cranial nerve that are affected by massage:

a) _____   e) _____

b) _____   f) _____

c) _____   g) _____

d) _____   h) _____

79. Match each of the following branches of the facial nerve with the muscle it affects:

_____ 1. posterior auricular nerve   A. the mouth
_____ 2. temporal nerve   B. the neck and the platysma muscle
_____ 3. zygomatic nerve   C. the chin and lower lip
_____ 4. buccal nerve   D. the temple, side of the forehead,
                                                     and upper part of the cheek
_____ 5. mandibular nerve   E. the ear at the base of the skull
_____ 6. cervical nerve   F. the temple, forehead, eyebrow,
                                                     and cheek

80. Identify the nerves in the head, face, and neck illustrated below:

1. _____
2. _____
3. _____
4. _____
5. _____
6. _____
7. _____
8. _____
9. _____
10. _____
11. _____
12. _____
13. _____
14. _____
15. _____
16. _____
17. _____
18. _____

81. The principal nerves supplying the superficial parts of the arm and hand are the _____,
_____ , _____ , and _____ .

82. Identify the nerves of the arm and hand illustrated below:

1. _____
2. _____
3. _____
4. _____

THE CIRCULATORY SYSTEM

83. The circulatory system, also referred to as the _____ or _____ system, controls the steady circulation of the blood through the body by means of the heart and blood vessels. It is made up of two divisions, the _____ consisting of the _____, _____, _____, and _____; and the _____ or _____ which acts as an aid to the blood system and consists of the _____, _____, _____, and other structures.

84. Which of the following is referred to as the body's pump?

    _____ a) cells

    _____ b) lungs

    _____ c) heart

    _____ d) veins

85. Match the following chambers of the heart with their descriptions:

    _____ 1. atrium

    _____ 2. ventricle

    _____ 3. valves

    A. lower, thick-walled chambers on the right and left ventricle

    B. structures between the chambers that allow the blood to flow in only one direction

    C. upper, thin-walled chambers on the right and left

86. Identify the parts of the heart illustrated below:

    1. _____

    2. _____

    3. _____

    4. _____

    5. _____

    6. _____

    7. _____

    8. _____

    9. _____

    10. _____

    11. _____

    12. _____

To upper part of body

87. The function of the blood vessels is to:

   _____ a) create nerve sensations

   _____ b) cleanse the body of impurities

   _____ c) transport blood to and from the heart

   _____ d) increase the oxygen supply to the lungs

88. The three categories of blood vessels are: _____ , _____ , and _____ .

89. What is blood?

_____

90. Match each of the following with its correct description:

   _____ 1. red blood cells   A. carries food and secretions to the cells and takes carbon dioxide away from the cells.

   _____ 2. hemoglobin   B. contribute to the blood clotting process

   _____ 3. white blood cells   C. a complex iron protein that gives the blood its bright red color

   _____ 4. platelets   D. destroy disease-causing germs

   _____ 5. plasma   E. carry oxygen to the body cells

91. Blood performs the following critical functions:

a) _____

b) _____

_____

c) _____

d) _____

_____

e) _____

92. The primary functions of the lymph vascular system are to:

a) _____

c) _____

c) _____

d) _____

93. The _____ arteries are the main sources of blood supply to the head, face, and neck.

    They are located on either side of the neck, and each one is divided into two branches called the

    _____ and the _____.

94. The _____ or _____ artery supplies blood to the lower region of

    the face, mouth, and nose. Some of its branches are:

    a) _____ which supplies blood to the chin and lower lip.

    b) _____ which supplies blood to the lower lip.

    c) _____ which supplies blood to the side of the nose.

    d) _____ which supplies blood to the upper lip and region of the nose.

95. The _____ artery is a continuation of the external carotid artery and supplies

    blood to the muscles of the front, side, and top of the head. Some of its important branches are:

    a) _____ which supplies blood to the forehead and upper eyelids.

    b) _____ which supplies blood to the side and crown of the head.

    c) _____ which supplies blood to the skin and masseter.

    d) _____ which supplies blood to the temples.

    e) _____ which supplies blood to the front part of the ear.

95. The blood returning to the heart from the head, face, and neck flows on each side of the neck in two

    principal veins: the _____ and _____.

96. Identify the arteries of the head, face, and neck illustrated below.

1. _____

2. _____

3. _____

4. _____

5. _____

6. _____

7. _____

8. _____

9. _____

10. _____

11. _____

12. _____

13. _____

14. _____

15. _____

16. _____

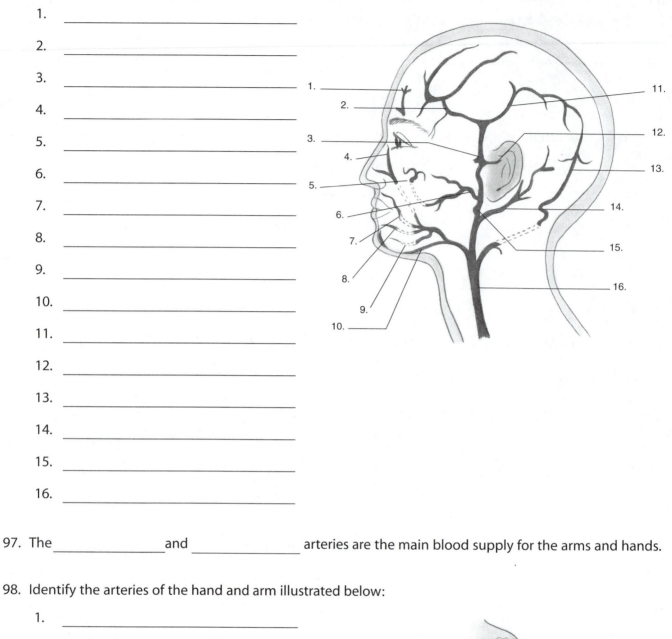

97. The _____ and _____ arteries are the main blood supply for the arms and hands.

98. Identify the arteries of the hand and arm illustrated below:

1. _____

2. _____

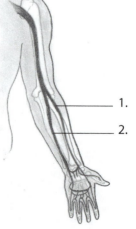

OTHER MAJOR SYSTEMS OF THE BODY

99. Match the name of the system with its description:

_____ 1. endocrine system   A. changes food into nutrients and waste

_____ 2. digestive system   B. enables breathing

_____ 3. excretory system   C. affects the growth, development, sexual activities, and health of the entire body

_____ 4. respiratory system   D. the skin and its various accessory organs

_____ 5. integumentary system   E. purifies the body by eliminating waste matter

100. What are glands?

_____

_____

101. Name the two main types of glands and their function:

a) _____

b) _____

_____

102. Match each organ with its function in the excretory system:

_____ 1. kidneys   A. eliminates decomposed and undigested food

_____ 2. liver   B. excrete urine

_____ 3. skin   C. exhale carbon dioxide

_____ 4. large intestine   D. eliminates perspiration

_____ 5. lungs   E. discharges bile

103. Identify the structures of the respiratory system illustrated below:

1. _____

2. _____

3. _____

4. _____

7
BASICS OF CHEMISTRY AND ELECTRICITY

Date: _____

Rating:_____

Text Pages: 167-198

POINT TO PONDER

"Get over the idea that only children should spend their time in study. Be a student so long as you still have something to learn, and this will mean all your life."—Henry L. Doherty

CHEMISTRY

1. _____ is the science that deals with the composition, structures and properties of

    matter, and how matter changes under different chemical conditions.

2. _____ is the study of substances that contain carbon.

3. _____ is the branch of chemistry dealing with compounds lacking carbon.

4. Match each of the following with its correct description:

    _____ 1. matter   A. the simplest form of matter
    _____ 2. element   B. the structural units that make up the elements
    _____ 3. atoms   C. formed by joining two or more atoms chemically
    _____ 4. molecule   D. any substance that occupies space, exists as a solid, liquid, or gas

5. Elemental molecules contain only one atom of the same element that are united chemically.

    _____ True

    _____ False

6. Compound molecules are chemical combinations of two or more atoms of the same elements.

    _____ True

    _____ False

7. All matter exists in one of three different physical forms: _____ , _____ , or _____ .

    These three forms are called the _____ . Matter assumes one of these states

    depending on its _____ .

8. Match the three different states of matter with their corresponding characteristics:

    _____ 1. solids   A. have a definite volume and weight but not a definite shape
    _____ 2. liquids   B. do not have a definite volume or shape
    _____ 3. gases   C. have a definite shape, volume, and weight

9. _____ are those characteristics that can be determined without a chemical reaction

    and that do not cause a chemical change in the identity of the substance. Physical properties include

    _____ .

10. _____ are those characteristics that can only be determined with a chemical

    reaction and that cause a chemical change in the identity of the substance.

11. What is oxidation?

    _____

12. Match the following change with its correct description:

    _____ 1. temporary hair color   A. a chemical change
    _____ 2. permanent hair color   B. a physical change

13. A pure substance is matter with no fixed chemical composition, definite proportions, and distinct properties.

    _____ True

    _____ False

14. The properties of chemical compounds are _____ the properties of the elements from

    which they were made.

15. In a _____ , each substance holds on to its own identity and its own distinct properties.

16. Solutions, suspensions, and emulsions are different types of _____ mixtures, all of which

    contain two or more different substances.

17. Match the following words with their description:

_____ 1. solution   A. a substance that dissolves another substance to form a solution
_____ 2. solute   B. a blended mixture of two or more solids, liquids, or gaseous substances
_____ 3. solvent   C. the dissolved substance in a solution

18. Water and oil are examples of:

_____ a) miscible liquids

_____ b) immiscible liquids

_____ c) flammable liquids

_____ d) nonflammable liquids

19. A _____ is a state in which solid particles are distributed throughout a liquid medium.

20. An _____ is a mixture of two or more immiscible substances united with the aid of a binder

or emulsifier.

21. _____ are substances that act as a bridge to allow oil and water to mix, or emulsify.

22. Mayonnaise is an example of an:

_____ a) oil-in-water emulsion of two immiscible liquids

_____ b) oil-in-water emulsion of two miscible liquids

_____ c) water-in-oil emulsion of two immiscible liquids

_____ d) water-in-oil emulsion of two miscible liquids

23. Match these common chemical ingredients used in salon products with their description:

_____ 1. alcohol   A. a colorless gas with a pungent odor, used to raise the pH in permanent waving, hair coloring, and lightening substances

_____ 2. alkanolamines   B. a readily evaporating, colorless liquid obtained by the fermentation of starch, sugar, and other carbohydrates

_____ 3. ammonia   C. two or more elements combined chemically that contain carbon and evaporate very quickly

_____ 4. glycerin   D. a special type of oil used in hair conditioners
_____ 5. silicones   E. a sweet, colorless, oily substance used as a solvent and a moisturizer
_____ 6. volatile organic F. substances used to neutralize acids or raise the pH of products
compounds

24. An ion is an

_____.

25. Ionization is the

_____.

26. An ion with a negative electrical charge is an _____ and an ion with a positive electrical

charge is a _____.

26. Without _____ there is no pH.

    a) oil

    b) cream

    c) water

    d) alcohol

27. The pH of water is:

    _____ a) 3

    _____ b) 5

    _____ c) 7

    _____ d) 9

28. The pH values are arranged on a scale ranging from 0 to 14. Match the following pH values with their

description:

    _____ 1. pH of 7   A. an alkaline solution

    _____ 2. pH of 3   B. a neutral solution

    _____ 3. pH of 12   C. an acidic solution

29. All _____ owe their chemical reactivity to the hydrogen ion (H^+). They have a pH below 7.0, taste

sour, and turn litmus paper from blue to red. They contract and harden the hair.

    a) acids

    b) alkalis

    c) emulsions

    d) surfactants

30. All_____ owe their chemical reactivity to the hydroxide (OH⁻) ion. They have a pH above 7.0, taste bitter, turn litmus paper from red to blue, and feel slippery and soapy on the skin. They soften and swell the hair.

    a) acids

    b) alkalis

    c) emulsions

    d) surfactants

31. Neutralizing shampoos and normalizing lotions used to neutralize hydroxide hair relaxers work by creating an acid-alkali _____ reaction.

32. _____ reactions are responsible for the chemical changes created by hair colors, hair lighteners, permanent wave solutions, and neutralizers.

33. _____ is a chemical reaction that combines an element or compound with oxygen to produce an oxide.

34. Chemical reactions that are characterized by or formed with the giving off of heat are called _____.

35. _____ is the rapid oxidation of any substance, accompanied by the production of heat and light.

36. Match each of the following with their descriptions:

    _____ 1. oxidized   A. contraction for reduction-oxidation
    _____ 2. reduced   B. chemical reaction caused when oxygen
                                            is subtracted from a substance
    _____ 3. reduction   C. when oxygen is subtracted from a substance
    _____ 4. oxidizing agent   D. when oxygen is combined with a substance
    _____ 5. redox   E. substance that releases oxygen

ELECTRICITY

37. _____ is a form of energy that, when in motion, exhibits magnetic, chemical, or thermal effects. It is a flow of electrons, which are negatively charged subatomic particles.

38. An _____ is the flow of electricity along a conductor.

39. Which of the following is a conductor?

    _____ a) wood

    _____ b) copper

    _____ c) cloth

    _____ d) alcohol

40. Which of the following is not an insulator?

    _____ a) rubber

    _____ b) silk

    _____ c) glass

    _____ d) water

41. A complete circuit is the path of an electric current from the generating source through insulators and

    back to its original source.

    _____ True

    _____ False

42. There are _____ types of electric current: _____ which is a constant,

    even-flowing current that travels in one direction only and produces a chemical reaction; and

    _____ which is a rapid and interrupted current, flowing first in one direction and

    then in the opposite direction.

43. Match the following words with their correct definitions:

    _____ 1. volt

    _____ 2. amp

    _____ 3. milliampere

    _____ 4. ohm

    _____ 5. watt

    A. unit that measures the strength of an electric current

    B. unit that measures $1/1000^{th}$ of an ampere

    C. unit that measures how much electric energy is being used in one second

    D. unit that measures the pressure that pushes the flow of electrons

    E. unit that measures the resistance of an electric current

44. The difference between a fuse and a circuit breaker is:

_____

_____

_____

_____

45. List all of the safety guidelines that you should adhere to when using electric appliances in the salon.

a) _____

b) _____

c) _____

d) _____

e) _____

f) _____

g) _____

_____

h) _____

i) _____

_____

j) _____

k) _____

l) _____

m) _____

n) _____

o) _____

ELECTROTHERAPY

46. Electronic facial treatments are commonly referred to as aromatherapy.

_____ True

_____ False

47. An_____ is an applicator for directing the electric current from the machine to the client's skin.

48. Unscramble the following words and use them to complete the sentences below.

    hodcate   odean   tlaripoy

    _____ indicates the negative or positive pole of an electric current. Electrotherapy devices

    always have one negatively charged pole and one positively charged pole. The positive electrode is

    called an_____ . It is usually red and is marked with a "P" or a plus (+) sign. The negative

    electrode is called a _____ . It is usually black and is marked with an "N" or a minus (-) sign.

49. The four main modalities used in cosmetology are:

    a) _____   c) _____

    b) _____   d) _____

50. Which polarity (negative or positive) of a galvanic current produces each of these chemical reactions:

    produces acidic reactions   _____
    softens tissues   _____
    hardens and firms tissues   _____
    closes the pores   _____
    opens the pores   _____
    stimulates and irritates the nerves _____
    contracts blood vessels   _____
    expands blood vessels   _____

51. _____ is the process of introducing water-soluble products into the skin with the use of

    electric current such as the use of the positive and negative poles of a galvanic machine.

52. _____ forces acidic substances into deeper tissues using galvanic current from the positive

    toward the negative pole.

53. _____ is the process of forcing liquids into the tissues from the negative toward the

    positive pole.

54. _____ is a process used to soften and emulsify grease deposits (oil) and blackheads in

    the hair follicles.

55. The faradic current is used during scalp and facial manipulations to cause muscular contractions that tone the facial muscles. Benefits derived from faradic current include:

a) _____   e) _____

b) _____   f) _____

c) _____   g) _____

d) _____

56. The sinusoidal current has the following advantages:

a) _____

b) _____

c) _____

57. The _____ current is a thermal or heat-producing current with a high rate of oscillation or vibration. It is commonly called the _____ and is used for both scalp and facial treatments.

58. The benefits from the use of Tesla high-frequency current are:

a) _____   d) _____

b) _____   e) _____

c) _____   f) _____

LIGHT THERAPY

59. Match the following words with their descriptions:

_____ 1. visible light   A. an invisible form of electromagnetic radiation
_____ 2. electromagnetic radiation   B. an electromagnetic radiation that is visible
_____ 3. wavelength   C. carries energy through space on waves
_____ 4. ultraviolet rays   D. distance between two successive peaks of energy

60. _____ are used to produce artificial light rays in the salon. These lamps are capable of producing the same rays that are produced by the sun.

61. _____ make up 5% of natural sunlight and are also referred to as _____

    or _____.

62. UV rays are applied with a lamp at a distance of _____ inches (76 to 91 cm). The therapy

    should begin with exposure times of _____ minutes with a gradual increase in exposure time

    to _____ minutes.

63. _____ make up 60% of natural sunlight, have long wavelengths, penetrate

    the deepest, and produce the most heat.

64. Infrared lamps should be operated at a distance of at least _____ inches (76 cm), for an exposure

    time of about _____ minutes.

65. _____ are the primary source of lights used for facial and scalp treatments.

66. The bulbs used for therapeutic visible light therapy are _____ , _____ , and _____.

67. The benefit of white light is:

    _____

68. The benefit of blue light is:

    _____

69. The benefit of red light is:

    _____

8
PROPERTIES OF THE HAIR AND SCALP

Date: _____

Rating:_____

Text Pages: 201-225

POINT TO PONDER:

"Knowledge is the eye of desire and can become the pilot of the soul."—Will Durant

STRUCTURE OF THE HAIR

1. The scientific study of hair, its diseases, and care is called _____.

2. Hair is part of the _____ , which is the largest and fastest-growing organ of the human body.

3. Full-grown human hair is divided into two parts: the hair _____ and the hair _____. The hair

   _____ is the part of the hair located below the surface of the scalp, and the hair _____ is the

   portion of the hair that projects beyond the skin.

4. Match the main structures of the hair root below with their description:

_____	1. follicle	A.	a small, cone-shaped elevation located at the base of the hair follicle
_____	2. hair bulb	B.	tubelike pocket in the skin or scalp that contains the hair root
_____	3. dermal papilla	C.	the lowest area; part of a hair strand
_____	4. arrector pili	D.	the oil glands of the skin, connected to the hair follicles
_____	5. sebaceous glands	E.	involuntary muscle fiber in the skin inserted in the base of the hair follicle

5. The sebaceous glands secrete an oily substance called_____, which lubricates the hair and skin.

6. Hair follicles are distributed all over the body, with the exception of the_____ and

   the _____.

7. What contains the blood and nerve supply that provides the nutrients needed for hair growth?

   _____ a) follicle

   _____ b) dermal papilla

   _____ c) sebaceous glands

   _____ d) hair bulb

8. Identify the parts of the skin and hair illustrated below.

   1. _____

   2. _____

   3. _____

   4. _____

   5. _____

   6. _____

   7. _____

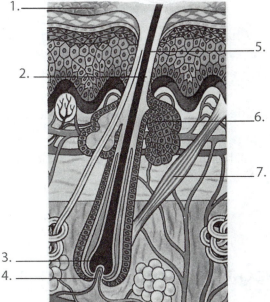

9. The three main layers of the hair shaft are the _____ , _____ , and _____ .

10. Describe the cuticle layer of hair.

_____

_____

11. Which if the following raises the cuticle layer of the hair and opens the space between the scales, which allows liquids to penetrate?

   _____ a) shrinking

   _____ b) swelling

   _____ c) defining

   _____ d) cutting

12. In order to penetrate the cuticle, oxidation haircolors, permanent waving solutions and chemical hair relaxers must have an acid pH to reach their target within the cortex.

_____ True

_____ False

13. The _____ is the middle layer of the hair, a fibrous protein core formed by elongated cells, containing melanin pigment.

14. What determines the elasticity and its natural color of the hair?

_____

15. The _____ is the innermost layer, sometimes referred to as the pith of the hair.

16. All hair has three layers—the cuticle, the cortex and the medulla.

_____ True

_____ False

THE CHEMICAL COMPOSITION OF HAIR

17. Hair is composed of _____ that grows from cells originating within the hair follicle.

18. The maturation of these cells is a process called _____ .

19. Hair is a living thing.

_____ True

_____ False

20. The elements that make up human hair are:

1. _____

2. _____

3. _____

4. _____

5. _____

21. Match the following terms with their description:

_____ 1. amino acids   A. the chemical bond that joins amino acids to each other

_____ 2. peptide bond   B. the units of structure in protein

_____ 3. polypeptide chain   C. the spiral shape of polypeptide chains when intertwined

_____ 4. helix   D. a long chain of amino acids linked by peptide bonds

22. Polypeptide chains are cross-linked together by three different types of side bonds called:

a) _____

b) _____

c) _____

23. Side bonds hold the hair fibers in place and account for the incredible _____ and _____ of human hair.

24. What kind of bond is a physical side bond that is easily broken by water or heat?

_____

25. What kind of a bond is a physical side bond that is broken by changes in pH?

_____

26. What kind of a bond is a chemical side bond that differs greatly from the kind of physical bonding seen in a hydrogen or salt bond?

_____

27. Disulfide bonds account for about _____ of the hair's overall strength.

28. All natural hair color is the result of the _____ located within the cortex.

29. If you have blonde hair which type of melanin do you mostly have? _____

30. If you have dark brown hair which type of melanin do you mostly have? _____

31. Gray hair is caused by the absence of _____.

32. The _____ of the hair refers to the amount of movement in the hair strand and is described as straight, wavy, curly, or extremely curly.

33. Wave pattern is always uniform on the head.

_____ True

_____ False

34. Match the following shape of hair's cross-section with the wave pattern most commonly associated with it:

_____ 1. round   A. extremely curly
_____ 2. oval   B. straight hair
_____ 3. flat   C. wavy hair

HAIR ANALYSIS

35. The **four** most important factors to consider in hair analysis are

_____ .

36. Match the following terms with their description:

_____ 1. texture   A. measures the number of individual hair strands on 1 square inch of scalp
_____ 2. density   B. the ability of the hair to absorb moisture
_____ 3. porosity   C. the ability of the hair to stretch and return to its original length without breaking
_____ 4. elasticity   D. the thickness or diameter of the individual hair strand

37. The average hair density is about _____ hairs per square inch.

38. Porous hair has a raised _____ layer that easily absorbs water.

39. Hair_____ is an indication of the strength of the side bonds that hold the hair's individual fibers in place.

40. Match the following terms with their description:

_____ 1. hair stream   A. tuft of hair that stands straight up
_____ 2. whorl   B. hair flowing in the same direction
_____ 3. cowlick   C. hair that forms in a circular pattern

41. Which of the following is *not* a cause of dry hair and scalp?

    _____ a) inactive sebaceous glands

    _____ b) active sebaceous glands

    _____ c) winter weather

    _____ d) desert climate

42. To treat dry hair and scalp you should use products that contain _____.

43. Oily hair and scalp is caused by _____ sebaceous glands and characterized by a greasy

    buildup on the scalp and an oily coating on the hair.

44. To treat oily hair and scalp you should_____shampoo.

HAIR GROWTH

45. The two main types of hair found on the body are _____ and _____ hair.

46. On adults, vellus is commonly found on the _____.

47. Terminal hair is commonly found on the _____.

48. Unscramble these words, then match them with their correct description:

    gloeten   neanag   agatecn

    _____   the growth phase of new hair

    _____   the brief transition period between the growth and
                                     resting phases of a hair follicle

    _____   the resting phase, the final phase in the hair cycle

49. What is the average growth of healthy scalp hair per month?

    _____ a) 1/4 inch

    _____ b) 1/2 inch

    _____ c) 1 inch

    _____ d) 2 inches

50. Shaving, clipping, and cutting the hair makes it grow back faster, darker, and coarser.

    _____ True

    _____ False

51. Scalp massage increases hair growth.

_____ True

_____ False

52. Gray hair is not coarser or more resistant than pigmented hair.

_____ True

_____ False

53. The amount of natural curl is not determined by racial background.

_____ True

_____ False

HAIR LOSS

54. It is normal to lose some hair every day.

_____ True

_____ False

55. Abnormal hair loss is called _____.

56. What happens during androgenic or androgenetic alopecia?

_____

_____

57. In men, androgenic alopecia is known as _____ and usually progresses to the

familiar horseshoe-shaped fringe of hair.

58. _____ is characterized by the sudden falling out of hair in round patches or baldness in

spots and may occur on the scalp and elsewhere on the body.

59. What causes alopecia areata?

_____

_____

60. _____ is temporary hair loss experienced at the conclusion of a pregnancy.

61. Name the only two products that have been proven to stimulate hair growth and are approved by the Food and Drug Administration (FDA) for that purpose.

_____

62. What is Minoxidil and how is it applied?

_____

63. What is Finasteride?

_____

64. Describe a surgical treatment for hair loss.

_____

_____

_____

65. What nonmedical options can hairstylists offer to counter hair loss?

_____

DISORDERS OF THE HAIR

66. _____ is the technical term for gray hair.

67. How many types of canities are there? Name them.

_____

68. _____ canities exists at or before birth. It occurs in albinos and occasionally in individuals with normal hair.

69. _____ canities develops with age and is the result of genetics.

70. What is ringed hair?

_____

_____

71. _____ or _____ is a condition of abnormal growth of hair.

72. List treatments for hypertrichosis:

  a) _____   d) _____

  b) _____   e) _____

  c) _____   f) _____

73. _____ is the technical term for split ends.

74. What are the treatments for trichoptilosis?

  a) _____

  b) _____

75. _____, or knotted hair, is characterized by brittleness and the formation of nodular

swellings along the hair shaft.

76. How should trichorrhexis nodosa be treated?

  _____

77. _____ is the technical term for beaded hair.

78. _____ is the technical term for brittle hair.

DISORDERS OF THE SCALP

79. Just as the skin on other parts of the body is continually being shed and replaced, the uppermost layer of the scalp is also being cast off and replaced.

  _____ True

  _____ False

80. What is dandruff?

  _____

81. What is the medical term for dandruff?

  _____

82. What are the suspected causes of dandruff?

a) _____

b) _____

c) _____

d) _____

e) _____

f) _____

83. What are the treatments for dandruff?

_____

_____

84. _____ is the technical term for scalp inflammation marked by dry dandruff, thin scales, and an itchy scalp.

85. _____ is a scalp inflammation marked by fatty (greasy or waxy) types of dandruff.

86. Dandruff is not contagious.

_____ True

_____ False

87. _____ is the medical term for ringworm.

88. What does tinea look like?

_____

89. Ringworm is caused by _____.

90. _____ is commonly known as ringworm of the scalp.

91. _____ is characterized by dry, sulfur-yellow, cuplike crusts on the scalp.

92. _____ is a highly contagious skin disease caused by the itch mite burrowing under

the skin.

93. _____ is the infestation of the hair and scalp with head lice.

94. A _____ , or boil, is an acute, localized bacterial infection of the hair follicle that produces

constant pain.

95. A _____ is an inflammation of the subcutaneous tissue caused by staphylococci.

DISCUSSION QUESTIONS

Answer the questions below and be prepared to discuss them in class at the appropriate time.

96. How does your hair define you? What does your hair style, color and length say about who you are and
the image you want to project to the outside world?

_____

97. Describe the emotional impact of hair loss on men.

_____

98. Describe the emotional impact of hair loss on women.

_____

9

PRINCIPLES OF HAIR DESIGN

Date: _____

Rating:_____

Text Pages: 227-252

POINT TO PONDER:

"Real intelligence is a creative use of knowledge, not merely the accumulation of facts."—D. Kenneth Winebrenner

PHILOSOPHY OF DESIGN

1. What is the first thing a good designer visualizes when beginning a project?

   _____

2. What is the first step in the creative process?

   _____

3. List some sources of inspiration.

   _____

   _____

4. What things, people or places inspire your creativity?

   _____

5. Once you have been inspired, what is the next step?

   _____

6. What is a hair designer's "trained eye"?

   _____

   _____

7. Having a strong foundation in technique and skills will allow you to take calculated _____ .

8. What is a "cookie cutter" hairdresser?

_____

_____

ELEMENTS OF HAIR DESIGN

9. The five basic elements of hair design are:

   1. _____

   2. _____

   3. _____

   4. _____

   5. _____

10. _____ is the outline of the overall hairstyle as seen from all angles. It is three-dimensional and changes as it is viewed from different angles.

11. The_____ is typically the aspect of the overall design that a client will react to first.

12. The hair form should be in proportion to the shape of the head and face, the length and width of the neck, and the shoulder line.

      _____ True

      _____ False

13. _____ is the area that the hairstyle occupies, also thought of as the area inside the form.

14. Space may also be called _____ . It is three-dimensional, having length, width, and depth.

15. _____ create the form, design, and movement of a hairstyle. They can be straight or curved.

16. Match the four basic types of lines with their description:

    _____ 1. horizontal lines   A. large or small, a full circle or just part of a circle
    _____ 2. vertical lines   B. positioned between horizontal and vertical lines
    _____ 3. diagonal lines   C. extending in the same direction and maintaining a
                                                   constant distance apart
    _____ 4. curved lines   D. straight up and down

17. Match the four basic types of lines with their usage:

    _____ 1. horizontal lines   A. soften a design
    _____ 2. vertical lines   B. can emphasize or minimize facial features
    _____ 3. diagonal lines   C. create length in hair design
    _____ 4. curved lines   D. creates width in hair design

18. Describe a single-line hairstyle.

    _____

19. Describe repeating lines in a hairstyle.

    _____

    _____

20. Describe contrasting lines in a hairstyle.

    _____

    _____

21. Describe transitional lines in a hairstyle.

    _____

22. _____ can be used to make all or part of the design appear larger or smaller.

23. Color can tie the _____ together.

24. _____ and_____ create the illusion of volume.

25. _____ and_____ colors recede or move in toward the head, creating the illusion of less volume.

26. How is the illusion of dimension, or depth, created?

    _____

27. Using a _____ color, you can draw a line in the hairstyle in the direction you want the eye

    to travel in.

28. Hair color must contrast with skin tone.

    _____ True

    _____ False

29. Straight hair reflects light better than other wave patterns.

    _____ True

    _____ False

30. Wave patterns can be created _____ with the use of heat or wet styling techniques.
    a) permanently
    b) temporarily

31. Chemical wave pattern changes are considered _____.
    a) permanent
    b) temporary

32. _____ wave patterns accent the face and are particularly useful when you wish to narrow a
    round head shape.

33. _____ wave patterns take attention away from the face and can be used to soften square or
    rectangular features.

PRINCIPLES OF HAIR DESIGN

34. The five part principles important for hair design are:

    1. _____

    2. _____

    3. _____

    4. _____

    5. _____

35. _____ is the harmonious relationship between parts or things, or the

    comparative relation of one thing to another.

36. When choosing a style for a woman with large hips or broad shoulders, you should create a style with
    volume.

    _____ True

    _____ False

37. When designing a hairstyle, hair may be as wide as you think will suit the client.

    _____ True

    _____ False

38. _____ means harmony or proportion; in hairstyling, it signifies the proper degree

    of height and width.

39. In _____ the design is similar on both sides of the face.

40. _____ features unequal proportions designed to balance facial features.

41. _____ is the regular, recurrent pattern of movement in a hairstyle.

42. Which of the following signifies a fast rhythm?

_____ a) tight curls

_____ b) loose curls

43. The _____ in a hairstyle is the place that the eye turns to first before traveling to the rest of the design.

44. You can create emphasis in hair styling by using:

a) _____

b) _____

c) _____

d) _____

45. _____ is the orderly and pleasing arrangement of shapes and lines and is the most important of the art principles.

CREATING HARMONY BETWEEN HAIRSTYLE AND FACIAL STRUCTURE

46. The professional's job is to downplay a client's best features and to accentuate those features that do not add to the person's attractiveness.

_____ True

_____ False

47. An artistic and suitable hairstyle takes into account the following characteristics of the client:

a) _____

b) _____

c) _____

48. What are the two main characteristics of hair type?

_____

49. Match each the following hair textures with its description:

_____ 1. fine, straight hair

_____ 2. straight, medium hair

_____ 3. straight, coarse hair

_____ 4. wavy, fine hair

_____ 5. wavy, medium hair

_____ 6. wavy, coarse hair

_____ 7. curly, fine hair

_____ 8. curly, medium hair

_____ 9. curly, coarse hair

_____ 10. very curly, fine hair

_____ 11. extremely curly, medium hair

_____ 12. extremely curly, coarse hair

A. can get very wide, rather than longer, as it grows

B. could separate and reveal too much of the client's scalp

C. will be extremely wide without proper maintenance

D. creates a wide silhouette, and looks romantic if left natural

E. generally best left short, otherwise too voluminous.

F. needs lots of heavy styling product to weight it down for styling

G. hard to curl but responds well to thermal styling

H. most versatile hair texture

I. lots of volume, difficult to maintain at home.

J. can be fragile; may appear fuller with a layered cut and style

K. hugs the head shape due, no body or volume

L. very versatile, has a good amount of movement

50. A client's facial shape is determined by the _____ and _____ of the facial bones.

51. The seven basic facial shapes are:

   1. _____

   2. _____

   4. _____

   5. _____

   6. _____

   7. _____

   8. _____

52. When designing a style for your client's facial type, you generally try to create the illusion of an _____ shaped face.

53. The face can be divided into three zones: _____

   _____ .

54. Describe the contours of the oval shaped face: _____

_____

55. Describe the contours of the round shaped face: _____

56. Describe the contours of the square shaped face: _____

_____

57. Describe the contours of the triangular shaped face: _____

58. Describe the contours of the oblong shaped face: _____

59. Describe the contours of the diamond shaped face: _____

_____

60. Describe the contours of the inverted triangle shaped face: _____

61. Match the face shape below with its most suitable hairstyle:

_____ 1. round   A. style the hair close to the head with no volume

_____ 2. square   B. keep hair close on top of head, add volume on sides

_____ 3. triangular   C. fullness across the jaw line and forehead, close at the cheekbone

_____ 4. oblong   D. soften hair at temples and jaw, add width around the ear area

_____ 5. diamond   E. a hairstyle that has height on top but is close at the sides

_____ 6. inverted Triangle   F. volume at the temples and some height at the top

62. If a client has a wide forehead you should style the hair _____.

63. If a client has a narrow forehead you should style hair _____.

64. If a client has close-set eyes you should style hair _____.

65. If a client has wide-set eyes you should style hair _____ .

66. If a client has a crooked nose you should style hair _____

_____ .

67. If a client has a wide, flat nose you should style hair _____

_____ .

68. If a client has a long, narrow nose you should style hair _____ .

69. If a client has a round jaw, style the hair with _____ .

70. If a client has a square jaw, style the hair with _____ .

71. If a client has a long jaw, style the hair with _____

_____ .

72. The _____ is the outline of the face, head, or figure seen in a side view.

73. Match the following basic profiles with their descriptions:

_____ 1. straight	A. has a prominent forehead and chin, with other features receded inward
_____ 2. convex	B. does not curve in or out dramatically, has only a very slight curvature
_____ 3. concave	C. has a receding forehead and chin

74. How should you style the hair for a receding forehead?

_____

75. How should you style the hair for a large forehead?

_____

76. How should you style the hair for a small nose?

_____

77. How should you style the hair for a prominent nose?

_____

78. How should you style the hair for a receding chin?

_____

79. How should you style the hair for a small chin?

_____

80. How should you style the hair for a large chin?

_____

81. If you determine that a client's head shape isn't perfectly rounded, what should you do?

_____

_____

82. What is the major consideration when creating a hairstyle for someone who wears glasses?

_____

_____

83. Name the ways that a fringe (bangs) can be parted.

_____

84. _____ are used to direct hair across the top of the head. They help develop height on top and make thin hair appear fuller.

85. _____ are used for an oval face, but also give an oval illusion to wide and round faces.

86. _____ are used to create the illusion of width or height in a hairstyle.

87. _____ create a dramatic effect.

DESIGNING FOR MEN

88. What things should be considered when selecting a style for a male client?

_____

89. In addition to making a fashion statement, what can a mustache or a beard be used for?

_____

90. A man who is balding with closely trimmed hair also could look very good in a closely groomed _____.

10

SHAMPOOING, RINSING, & CONDITIONING

Date: _____

Rating:_____

Text Pages: 255-279

POINT TO PONDER:

"I found that the harder I work, the more luck I seem to have."—Thomas Jefferson

1. What is the importance of a pleasant experience for the client during the shampoo?

   _____

   _____

2. The time spent on the shampoo can help the client relax and gives you time to _____

   _____.

3. A client with an infectious disease should not be treated in the salon and should be referred to a physician.

   _____ True

   _____ False

4. To be effective, a shampoo must remove all _____ ,_____ ,_____ , and

   _____ without adversely affecting either the scalp or hair.

5. How often should the scalp and hair be cleansed?

   _____

6. Oily hair should be shampooed more often than normal or dry hair.

   _____ True

   _____ False

UNDERSTANDING SHAMPOO

7. What is the best way to select a shampoo for a client?

_____

8. List the most commonly recognized hair types:

   a) _____   c) _____

   b) _____   d) _____

9. Virgin hair is hair that has not been _____

_____.

10. A shampoo that is more _____ can have a pH rating from 0 to 6.9.

11. A shampoo that is more _____ can have a pH rating from 7.1 to 14.

12. The _____ the pH rating, the stronger and harsher the shampoo is to the hair.

13. _____ is rain water or chemically softened water.

14. _____ contains certain minerals that lessen the ability of soap or shampoo to lather readily.

15. Soft water is preferred for shampooing.

   _____ True

   _____ False

16. A surfactant is a cleansing agent.

   _____ True

   _____ False

17. A surfactant molecule has two ends: a _____, or water-attracting, "head," and a

   _____, or oil-attracting, "tail."

18. During the shampooing process, the hydrophilic head attracts _____, and the lipophilic tail

   attracts _____.

19. Match the type of shampoo below with its purpose for use:

_____ 1. acid-balanced shampoos

A. cleanse the hair and cut through product buildup

_____ 2. conditioning shampoos

B. cleanse the hair while keeping it at the pH of the skin

_____ 3. medicated shampoos

C. cleanse the hair while making it smooth and shiny

_____ 4. clarifying shampoos

D. cleanse the hair while relieving scalp conditions

_____ 5. balancing shampoos

E. cleanse the hair without the use of soap and water

_____ 6. dry or powder shampoos

F. cleanse hair and brighten hair color

_____ 7. color-enhancing shampoos

G. cleanse and wash away excess oiliness

CONDITIONERS

20. _____ are special chemical agents applied to the hair to deposit protein or moisturizer, to

help restore its strength and give it body, or to protect it against possible breakage.

21. Conditioners are valuable because they: _____

_____

_____ .

23. Match the type of conditioner below with its function:

_____ 1. Rinse-through

A. a deep, penetrating conditioner, left on the hair for 10 to 20 minutes

_____ 2. Treatment

B. applied to the hair and not rinsed out before styling

_____ 3. Leave-in

C. a finishing rinse used in detangling

24. What is a humectant?

_____

25. An_____ usually remains on the hair for a very short period of time and contain

humectants to improve the appearance of dry, brittle hair.

26. Heavier and creamier than instant conditioners, _____ also have a longer application time

(10 to 20 minutes) and contain many of the same ingredients as instant conditioners but are formulated

to be more penetrating and to have longer staying power.

27. _____ are designed to slightly increase hair diameter with a coating action,

thereby adding body to the hair.

28. How do protein conditioners work?

_____

_____

29. _____ , also known as hair masks or conditioning packs, are chemical

mixtures of concentrated protein in the heavy cream base of a moisturizer.

30. Match each of the following conditioning agents with its description:

_____ 1. spray-on thermal protectors   A. soften and improve the health of the scalp
_____ 2. scalp conditioners   B. promote healing of the scalp
_____ 3. medicated scalp lotions   C. remove oil accumulation from the scalp
_____ 4. scalp astringent lotions   D. applied to hair prior to thermal service
                                                     for protection

BRUSHING THE HAIR

31. List three reasons brushing is good for the hair and scalp.

a) _____

b) _____

c) _____

32. You should always brush a client's hair prior to shampoo in preparation for every service.

_____ True

_____ False

11

HAIRCUTTING

See Milady's Standard Cosmetology Practical Workbook

12

HAIRSTYLING

See Milady's Standard Cosmetology Practical Workbook

13

BRAIDING AND BRAID EXTENSIONS

See Milady's Standard Cosmetology Practical Workbook

14

WIGS AND HAIR ENHANCEMENTS

See Milady's Standard Cosmetology Practical Workbook

15

CHEMICAL TEXTURE SERVICES

Date: _____

Rating: _____

Text Pages: 485–543

POINT TO PONDER:

"Anyone who stops learning is old, whether this happens at twenty or eighty. Anyone who keeps on learning not only remains young, but becomes constantly more valuable regardless of physical capacity."— Harvey Ullman

1. _____ cause a chemical change that permanently alters the natural wave

   pattern of the hair.

2. Texture services can be used to _____ straight hair, _____ extremely curly hair, or

   _____ coarse, straight hair and make it more pliable and easier to work with.

3. Texture services include _____ , _____ , and _____

   _____ .

THE STRUCTURE OF HAIR

4. The outer layer of the hair, called the _____ , surrounds the inner layers and protects the hair

   from damage.

5. A strong, compact cuticle layer makes the hair _____ , meaning that the hair resists

   penetration and is more difficult to service.

6. How do chemical hair texturizers change the hair's natural curl pattern?

   _____

   _____

7. Coarse, resistant hair with a strong, compact cuticle layer requires a texturizer, which is highly acidic.

_____ True

_____ False

8. The polypeptide chains of the cortex are connected by end bonds and cross-linked by side bonds that form the fibers and structure of hair. These chemical bonds hold the hair in its natural _____ and are responsible for the _____ of human hair.

9. Changing the natural wave pattern of the hair involves breaking the _____.

10. The chemical bonds that join the amino acids are called _____ or _____.

11. The peptide bonds, in turn, link together to form long chains of amino acids called _____ _____.

12. _____ are long, coiled, complex polypeptide chains made of many different amino acids linked together, end-to-end, like pop beads.

13. Name the three types of side bonds, or cross bonds: _____.

14. What makes wet setting, thermal styling, permanent waving, soft curl permanents, and chemical hair relaxing possible?

_____

15. _____ are formed between two cysteine amino acids, located on neighboring polypeptide chains.

16. A disulfide bond joins a cysteine sulfur atom on one polypeptide chain with a second cysteine sulfur atom on a neighboring polypeptide chain to form _____ , the oxidized form of cysteine.

17. Disulfide bonds are weak chemical side bonds that are broken by heat or water.

_____ True

_____ False

18. Which bonds are the strongest of the three side bonds?

_____

19. Salt bonds are relatively _____ physical side bonds that are the result of an attraction

between opposite electrical charges.

20. Salt bonds are not easily broken by changes in pH, as in permanent waving, and do not re-form when the pH returns to normal.

_____ True

_____ False

21. Salt bonds account for how much of the hair's total strength?

_____ a) Half

_____ b) Two-thirds

_____ c) One-third

_____ d) Three-quarters

22. Hydrogen bonds are relatively weak physical side bonds that are the result of an attraction between opposite electrical charges.

_____ True

_____ False

23. Hydrogen bonds are easily broken by water, as in wet setting, or heat, as in thermal styling, and re-form as the hair dries or cools.

_____ True

_____ False

24. Hydrogen bonds account for how much of the hair's total strength?

_____ a) Half

_____ b) Two-thirds

_____ c) One-third

_____ d) Three-quarters

25. A wet set is an example of a _____ change that results from breaking and re-forming the hydrogen bonds within the hair.

26. Thermal styling with hair dryers, curling irons, and pressing combs are examples of chemical change that involve permanent results.

   _____ True

   _____ False

THE CLIENT CONSULTATION

27. List the topics to cover in the client consultation prior to a chemical texture service:

   a) _____

   b) _____

   c) _____

   d) _____

   _____

   e) _____

   _____

   f) _____

   g) _____

28. Client records should include a complete evaluation of the _____ _____ of the hair prior to the service, and the results that are expected. Extra caution should be used to determine any previous problems or _____ the client may have had in the past.

29. It is okay to proceed with chemical texture services if there are minor skin abrasions or scalp disease.

   _____ True

   _____ False

30. The five most important factors to consider in hair analysis are _____

   _____ .

31. Match the following hair textures with the phrase that best describes it:

   _____ 1. coarse hair   A. fragile, easy to process, easier to damage from perm services
   _____ 2. medium hair   B. requires more processing and may be more resistant to processing
   _____ 3. fine hair   C. considered normal and does not pose any special problems or concerns

32. _____ measures the number of strands of hair on the head, indicating how thick

   or thin the hair is.

33. _____ is the ability of the hair to absorb moisture.

34. Match the following degree of porosity with its description:

   _____ 1. resistant hair   A. easily absorbs solution
   _____ 2. normal porosity   B. has a compact cuticle layer that resists penetration
   _____ 3. porous hair   C. neither resistant nor overly porous

35. _____ is an indication of the strength of the side bonds that hold the individual

   fibers of the hair in place.

36. More than any other single factor, the _____ of the hair determines its ability to hold curl.

37. Wet hair with normal elasticity can stretch up to what percent of its original length?

   _____ a) 10
   _____ b) 25
   _____ c) 50
   _____ d) 75

38. The individual growth direction of the hair causes _____

   that influence the finished hairstyle and must be considered when selecting the base direction and

   wrapping pattern for each permanent wave.

PERMANENT WAVING

40. Permanent waving is a two-step process.

    _____ True

    _____ False

41. In permanent waving, the size, shape, and type of curl are determined by the permanent wave solution chosen.

    _____ True

    _____ False

42. Once in the cortex, the waving solution breaks the disulfide bonds through a chemical reaction called

    _____.

43. The reduction reaction in permanent waving is due to the addition of _____.

44. The reducing agents used in permanent waving solutions are _____ compounds.

45. _____ is a colorless liquid with a strong unpleasant odor and provides

    the hydrogen that causes the reduction reaction in permanent waving solutions.

46. The addition of ammonia to thioglycolic acid produces a new chemical called _____

    _____ , which is alkaline.

47. Alkaline waves process at:

    _____ a) high heat

    _____ b) room temperature

    _____ c) freezing

    _____ d) below zero

48. Acid waves process at:

_____ a) heated temperature

_____ b) room temperature

_____ c) freezing temperature

_____ d) below-zero temperature

49. _____ is the main active ingredient in acid waves, which have a low pH.

50. How do acid-balanced waves process?

_____

51. _____ create an exothermic chemical reaction that heats up the

perming solution and speeds up the processing.

52. Which of the following must be added to exothermic waves in order for them to process?

_____ a) waving solution

_____ b) an activator

_____ c) a neutralizer

_____ d) water

53. Mixing an oxidizer with the permanent waving solution causes_____

_____

_____.

54. _____ are activated by an outside heat source, usually a conventional

hood-type hair dryer.

55. _____ use an ingredient that does not evaporate as readily as

ammonia, so there is very little odor associated with their use.

56. _____ use an ingredient other than ammonium thioglycolate as the

primary reducing agent.

57. The use of sulfates, sulfites, and bisulfites presents an alternative to ammonium thioglycolate known as

_____ .

58. The strength of any permanent wave is based on the concentration of its _____ .

59. In permanent waving, most of the processing takes place as soon as the solution _____

_____ , within the first five to ten minutes.

60. When does over processing usually occur?

_____

61. Resistant hair may not become completely saturated with just one application of waving solution.

_____ True

_____ False

62. What occurs if the hair is under processed?

_____

63. _____ is the process of stopping the action of a permanent wave solution and

hardening the hair in its new form by the application of a chemical solution called the neutralizer.

64. The two important functions of neutralization are:

a) _____

b) _____

65. The most common neutralizer is _____ .

66. In a properly processed permanent wave the bonds in the hair are re-formed:

_____ a) temporarily

_____ b) immediately

_____ c) continuously

_____ d) accurately

67. Some home hair coloring products contain_____ that are not compatible with

    permanent waving and leave a coating on the hair that may cause _____

    _____.

CHEMICAL HAIR RELAXERS

68. _____ is the process of rearranging the basic structure of extremely curly

    hair into a straight form.

69. The chemistry of thio relaxers and permanent waving is exactly the same.

    _____ True

    _____ False

70. The two most common types of chemical hair relaxers are_____

    and _____.

71. Extremely curly hair grows in long twisted spirals or coils, with the thinnest and weakest sections of the
    hair strands located at their twists.

    _____ True

    _____ False

72. _____ usually have a pH above 10 and a higher concentration of ammonium

    thioglycolate than is used in permanent waving.

73. The_____ used with thio relaxers is an oxidizing agent, usually hydrogen peroxide,

    just as in permanents.

74. The_____ is the active ingredient in all hydroxide relaxers.

75. No hydroxide relaxers are capable of swelling the hair up to twice its normal diameter.

    _____ True

    _____ False

76. Hydroxide relaxers are not compatible with thio relaxers.

    _____ True

    _____ False

77. Hydroxide relaxers remove one atom of sulfur from a disulfide bond, converting it into a lanthionine

    bond by a process called _____.

78. The neutralization of hydroxide relaxers involves oxidation.

    _____ True

    _____ False

79. What does the application of an acid-balanced shampoo or a normalizing lotion do?

    _____

80. _____ are ionic compounds formed by a metal—sodium (Na), potassium (K),

    or lithium (Li)—which is combined with oxygen (O) and hydrogen (H).

81. Sodium hydroxide relaxers are commonly called _____.

82. _____ and _____ relaxers are often advertised and

    sold as "no mix-no lye" relaxers.

83. Guanidine straightens hair completely with much less scalp irritation than other hydroxide relaxers.

    _____ True

    _____ False

84. _____ and _____ are sometimes used as low-pH hair relaxers.

85. Sulfites are marketed as mild alternative relaxers and completely straighten extremely curly hair.

    _____ True

    _____ False

86. _____ is an oily cream used to protect the skin and scalp during hair relaxing.

87. _____ require the application of base cream to the entire scalp prior to the

    application of the relaxer.

88. _____ do not require application of a protective base because they contain a

    base cream that is designed to melt at body temperature.

89. Match the strength of the relaxer with the hair type it is formulated for:

    _____ 1. mild strength   A. formulated for maximum straightening extremely curly
    _____ 2. regular strength   B. formulated for fine, color-treated, or damaged hair
    _____ 3. super strength   C. formulated for normal hair texture with a medium natural curl

SOFT CURL PERMANENTS

90. _____ do not straighten the hair; they simply make the existing curl larger

    and looser.

91. A soft curl permanent is a combination of a _____ and a _____

    _____.

92. Soft curl permanents use _____ and oxidation neutralizers, just as thio

    permanent waves do.

16

HAIRCOLORING

Date: _____

Rating:_____

Text Pages: 545–602

POINT TO PONDER:

"The young [person] who has the combination of the learning of books with the learning which comes of doing things with the hands need not worry about getting along in the world today or at any time."—William S. Knudsen

1. _____ is both a science and an art.

2. A skilled hair colorist needs to become an expert in the following processes:

   a) _____

   b) _____

   c) _____

   d) _____

WHY PEOPLE COLOR THEIR HAIR

3. The most common reasons clients color their hair are:

   a) _____

   b) _____

   c) _____

   d) _____

   e) _____

COLOR THEORY

4. Color is a form of_____.

5. The_____ is a system for understanding color relationships.

6. The Law of Color states: When combining colors, you will always get the same result from the same combination.

   _____ True

   _____ False

7. _____are pure or fundamental colors that cannot be achieved from a mixture.

8. The primary colors are:

   _____.

9. _____colors are created from the three primary colors.

   a) Some

   b) All

   c) Most

   d) A few

10. Colors with a pure dominance of blue are_____toned colors, and colors with a predominance of red are_____ toned colors.

11. _____is the darkest of the primary colors and is the only cool primary color.

12. _____is the medium primary color.

13. Red added to blue-based colors will cause them to appear_____.

    a) darker

    b) lighter

    c) trendier

    d) classic

14. Red added to yellow colors will cause them to become _____.

    a) darker

    b) lighter

    c) trendier

    d) classic

15. _____ is the lightest of the primary colors.

16. When you add yellow to other colors, the resulting color is _____ in appearance.

    a) deeper and darker

    b) lighter and brighter

    c) more youthful

    d) more sophisticated

17. When all three primary colors are present in equal proportions, the resulting color is _____.

18. A _____ is a color obtained by mixing _____ parts of two primary colors.

19. The secondary colors are:

    _____.

20. Green is an equal combination of _____.

21. Orange is an equal combination of _____.

22. Violet is an equal combination of _____.

23. A _____ is an intermediate color achieved by mixing a secondary color and its

    neighboring primary color on the color wheel in _____ amounts.

24. The tertiary colors include:

    _____.

25. Natural-looking hair color is made up of a combination of _____ colors.

26. _____ are a primary and secondary color positioned opposite each other on the color wheel.

27. Next to each color below, list its complementary color:

    blue   _____

    red   _____

    yellow   _____

28. Complementary colors _____ each other.

    a) coxidize

    b) neutralize

    c) brighten

    d) darken

29. Place a "P", "S", and "T" on the color wheel in their proper places to signify primary, secondary, and tertiary colors.

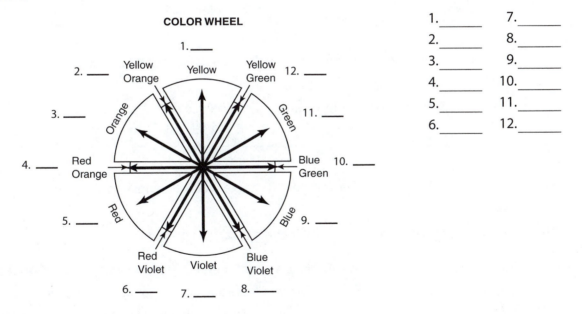

COLOR WHEEL

1. _____   7. _____
2. _____   8. _____
3. _____   9. _____
4. _____   10. _____
5. _____   11. _____
6. _____   12. _____

HAIR FACTS

30. The _____ of a client's hair is a determining factor in choosing which hair color to use.

31. Some hair color products may cause a dramatic change in the structure of the hair, while others cause relatively little change.

    _____ True

    _____ False

32. Name the three main parts of the hair:

a) _____

b) _____

c) _____

33. The cortex contains the natural pigment called _____, which determines natural hair color.

34. Hair texture is determined by the_____.

35. Large, medium, and small diameter hair strands translate into _____

hair textures respectively.

36. Match the following textures of hair with their ability to take hair color:

_____ 1. fine hair   A. average response to hair color products

_____ 2. medium-textured hair   B. takes longer to process

_____ 3. coarse-textured hair   C. takes color quickly

37. _____ is the number of hairs per square inch, ranging from thin to thick.

38. Why must hair density be taken into account when applying hair color?

_____

39. _____ hair accepts hair color faster and permits darker color than less porous hair.

40. Match the following degrees of porosity with their effect on the coloring process:

_____ 1. low porosity   A. hair is normal and processes in an average amount of time

_____ 2. average porosity   B. hair is overporous, takes color quickly, and fades quickly

_____ 3. high porosity   C. hair is resistant and requires a longer processing time

41. Name the two types of melanin in the cortex and what they do:

a) _____

b) _____

42. Natural hair color can be a combination of both types of melanin, called _____.

43. _____ is the pigment that lies under the natural hair color and must be taken

   into consideration when you select a hair color.

44. Generally, when you lighten natural hair color, you_____ contributing pigment.

   a) hide

   b) expose

   c) change

   d) alter

45. The foundation of hair coloring is based on modifying the_____ with hair color

   products to create new pigment.

THE LEVEL SYSTEM

46. _____ is the unit of measurement used to identify the lightness or darkness of a color; it is

   sometimes referred to as_____ or _____ .

47. Colorists use the Level System to analyze the_____ of a hair color.

48. Hair color levels are arranged on a scale of_____ , with 1 being the_____

   and 10 being the_____ .

49. The term_____ is used to describe the warmth or coolness of a color.

50. Common words that indicate warmth in hair color are:

   _____ .

51. Common words that indicate coolness in hair color are:

   _____ .

52. _____ refers to the strength of a color tone and is described as mild, medium, or strong.

53. Artificial hair colors are developed from the primary and secondary colors that form _____

which are the predominant tonality of an existing color.

54. What kind of color results will be delivered by each of the following?

    violet base color: _____

    blue base color: _____

    red-orange base color   _____

    gold base color   _____

55. Identifying _____ is the first step in performing a hair color service.

56. Name two tools that are most valuable in helping you determine hair color values:

    _____

57. Describe how to determine natural hair color level:

    a) _____

    _____

    b) _____

    _____

    c) _____

    _____

    d) _____

    _____

58. Gray hair is normally associated with _____ , although _____ is also a contributing

factor.

59. Once the hair begins to turn gray, it generally becomes completely white within a year.

    _____ True

    _____ False

60. People whose hair is characterized as "salt and pepper" have:

_____ a) too much sodium in their diet

_____ b) used an incorrect hair color formula

_____ c) too much pepper in their diet

_____ d) have a blend of dark hair and white hair

61. Match the following description with the percentage of gray it indicates:

_____ 1.	more pigmented than gray hair	A. 50%
_____ 2.	even mixture of gray and pigmented hair	B. 70% - 90%
_____ 3.	more gray than pigmented	C. 100%
_____ 4.	virtually no pigmented hair; tends to look white	D. 30%

TYPES OF HAIR COLOR

62. Name the four categories that hair coloring products generally fall into:

_____ .

63. All four hair color categories except for temporary color require a _____ before application to

determine if the client is allergic to the product.

64. _____ is a chemical process involving the diffusion of the natural color pigment or

artificial color from the hair.

65. All permanent hair color products and lighteners contain both a _____

and an _____ as part of their composition.

66. The role of the alkalizing ingredient is to:

a) _____

b) _____

c) _____

67. When the tint containing the alkalizing ingredient is combined with the developer, the peroxide

becomes alkaline and diffuses through the hair fiber, entering the _____ ,

where the melanin is located.

68. What action causes the hair to lighten?

_____

69. The pigment molecules in _____ are large and therefore do not penetrate the cuticle

layer, allowing only a coating action that may be removed by shampooing.

70. List products that provide temporary hair color:

a) _____

b) _____

c) _____

d) _____

e) _____

71. _____ is hair color formulated to last through several shampoos, depending

on the hair's porosity.

72. How does semi-permanent hair color work?

_____

_____

73. How long does does semipermanent hair color last?

_____ a) three to four shampoos

_____ b) six to eight shampoos

_____ c) ten to twelve shampoos

_____ d) permanently

74. How many shades does semi-permanent hair color lift?

_____ a) no lift

_____ b) two shades

_____ c) four shades

_____ d) six shades

75. Semi-permanent hair color is formulated without_____ and is generally as gentle to the hair as shampoo, but it does require a patch test before application.

76. Why do some semi-permanent hair colors require use of activators?

_____

_____

77. _____ is similar in nature to semi-permanent hair color but is longer lasting.

78. How many shades does demi-permanent hair color lift?

    _____ a) no lift

    _____ b) two shades

    _____ c) four shades

    _____ d) six shades

79. Demi-permanent hair colors are ideal for covering_____ hair, refreshing faded permanent color, depositing tonal changes without lift, corrective coloring, and reverse highlighting.

80. Demi-permanent is also called _____ hair color.

81. Demi-permanent hair color is available as a_____.

82. _____ is mixed with a developer (hydrogen peroxide) and remains in the hairshaft until the new growth of hair occurs.

83. Permanent hair color products generally contain _____.

84. Aniline derivatives are small compounds that can_____.

85. Permanent tint molecules are trapped within the_____ of the hair and cannot be shampooed out.

86. Permanent hair coloring products are regarded as the best products for covering _____ hair.

87. Permanent hair coloring simultaneously removes _____ from the hair through the

action of lightening while adding _____ to both the gray and the pigmented hair.

88. A _____ is an oxidizing agent that, when mixed with an oxidative hair color, supplies the

necessary oxygen gas to develop color molecules and create a change in hair color.

89. The pH of developer is:

_____ a) between 1.0 and 2.3

_____ b) between 2.5 and 4.5

_____ c) between 6.5 and 7.5

_____ d) between 8.5 and 9.5

90. Name the most commonly used developer on the market:

_____

91. _____ is the measure of the potential oxidation of varying strengths of hydrogen peroxide.

92. Match the following volumes of hydrogen peroxide with its common use:

1.____10 volume   A. used to achieve most results with permanent hair color and gray coverage
2.____20 volume   B. use when less lightening is desired
3.____30 volume   C. used with high-lift colors to provide maximum lift in a one-step service
4.____40 volume   D. used for additional lift with permanent hair color

93. _____ such as henna are natural colors obtained from the leaves

or bark of plants.

94. If a client has used natural hair colors it is fine to use chemical coloring products right over them.

_____ True

_____ False

95. _____ contain metal salts and change hair color gradually by progressive buildup

and exposure to air, creating a dull, metallic appearance.

96. Metallic hair colors have historically been marketed to:

_____ a) young women

_____ b) men

_____ c) teens

_____ d) older women

97. _____are the chemical compounds that lighten hair by dispersing, dissolving, and

decolorizing the natural hair pigment.

98. What happens when hydrogen peroxide is mixed into the lightener formula?

_____

99. Hair lighteners are used to:

a) _____

b) _____

c) _____

d) _____

e) _____

f) _____

100. How many stages of color does hair go through as it lightens?

_____ a) three

_____ b) five

_____ c) eight

_____ d) ten

101. Name the colors the hair goes through in the de-colorization process:

a) _____   f) _____

b) _____   g) _____

c) _____   h) _____

d) _____   i) _____

e) _____   j) _____

102. Why would a colorist choose to decolorize a client's hair before tinting?

_____

_____

103. _____ are semi-permanent, demi-permanent, and permanent hair color products that are used primarily on pre-lightened hair to achieve pale and delicate colors.

104. All hair will go through all 10 degrees of de-colorization.

_____ True

_____ False

105. How can you tell if you have damaged the hair during the decolorization process?

_____

CONSULTATION

106. The hair color consultation should include:

a) _____

_____

b) _____

_____

c) _____

_____

d) _____

_____

e) _____

_____

f) _____

_____

g) _____

107. List some questions you might ask the client during your consultation:

a) _____

b) _____

c) _____

d) _____

e) _____

108. A _____ is used by many salons when providing chemical services. Its purpose is to explain to clients that if their hair is in questionable condition, it may not withstand the requested chemical treatment.

109. When working with hair color, you will have to determine whether your clients have any allergies or sensitivities to the mixture. To do this you will administer a _____.

110. How many hours prior to application of aniline tint or toner should a patch test be given?

_____ a) 5 to 10

_____ b) 12 to 18

_____ c) 24 to 48

_____ d) 62 to 78

111. The tint used for the patch test must be _____

_____.

112. A negative skin test result will show:

_____.

113. A positive skin test result will show:

_____.

114. Permanent hair color applications are classified as either _____-process or _____-process.

115. _____ is a process that lightens and colors the hair in a single application.

116. Single-process tints usually contain:

a) _____   c) _____

b) _____   d) _____

117. _____ , also known as double-application tinting and two-step coloring, is a technique requiring two separate procedures in which the hair is pre-lightened before the depositing color is applied.

118. A _____ refers to the first time the hair is tinted.

119. List the four basic questions you should ask yourself when formulating a hair color:

a) _____

b) _____

c) _____

d) _____

120. The combination of the shade selected and the volume of hydrogen peroxide determines the _____ of a hair color.

121. What are the two main methods of applying permanent color?

_____

_____

122. How should you mix color in an applicator bottle?

_____

123. How should you mix color using a brush and bowl?

_____

_____

124. As the hair grows, you will need to _____ it to keep it looking attractive and to avoid a two-toned effect.

125. In a retouch, the tint should be applied to:

_____ a) the hair at the ends only

_____ b) the hair at the mid-shaft only

_____ c) the new growth only

_____ d) the pre-lightened hair only

126. A visible line separating colored hair from new growth is called:

_____ a) hyperpigmentation

_____ b) hypopigmentation

_____ c) line of demarcation

_____ d) line of decolorization

127. Prelightening is:

_____.

128. There are _____ steps in a pre-lightening procedure:

a) 1

b) 2

c) 3

d) 4

LIGHTENING TECHNIQUES

129. On-the-scalp lighteners, which can be used directly on the scalp, are available in what forms?

_____

130. Off-the-scalp lighteners, which cannot be used directly on the scalp, are available in what form?

_____

131. List the benefits of using oil and cream lighteners:

a) _____

b) _____

c) _____

132. Cream lighteners may be mixed with:

_____ a) darkeners

_____ b) brighteners

_____ c) activators

_____ d) stimulators

133. What does an activator do?

_____

134. How many activators can be used for on-the-scalp lightener applications?

_____ a) one

_____ b) two

_____ c) three

_____ d) four

135. How many activators can be used for off-the-scalp lightener applications?

_____ a) one

_____ b) two

_____ c) three

_____ d) four

136. Name the factors that affect processing time for lightening:

a) _____

b) _____

c) _____

d) _____

e) _____

137. To determine the processing time for your lightening service, the condition of the hair after lightening, and the end results, you should perform a _____.

138. A patch test is not necessary if the client is having toner applied after lightening.

_____ True

_____ False

139. _____ are used primarily on pre-lightened hair to achieve pale, delicate colors.

140. Name the two processes required for a double-process application:

a) _____

b) _____

141. After the hair goes through the 10 stages of de-colorizing, the color that is left in the hair is

known as its_____.

SPECIAL EFFECTS HAIR COLORING

142. Special effects hair coloring refers to any technique that involves _____.

143. Coloring some of the hair strands lighter than the natural color to add the illusion of sheen and depth is
called _____.

144. Coloring strands of hair darker than the natural color is called _____.

145. Name the three most frequently used techniques for achieving highlights:

a) _____

b) _____

c) _____

146. The_____ involves pulling clean strands of hair through a perforated cap with a thin

plastic or metal hook.

147. The_____ of strands pulled through determines the degree of highlighting or lowlighting

you can achieve.

148. The_____ involves coloring selected strands of hair by slicing or weaving out sections, placing them on foil or plastic wrap, applying lightener or color, and sealing them in the foil or plastic wrap.

149. _____ involves taking a narrow, 1/8" section of hair by making a straight part at the scalp, positioning the hair over the foil, and applying lightener or color. In _____ , selected strands are picked up from a narrow section of hair with a zigzag motion of the comb, and lightener or color is applied only to these strands.

150. The_____ technique involves the painting of a lightener (usually powder lightener) directly onto clean, styled hair.

151. To avoid affecting untreated hair, you may choose:

a) _____

b) _____

c) _____

152. _____ are prepared by combining permanent hair color, hydrogen peroxide, and shampoo.

153. When should you use a highlighting shampoo tint?

_____

154. _____ are a mixture of shampoo and hydrogen peroxide and slightly lighten the natural color.

SPECIAL PROBLEMS IN HAIR COLOR/CORRECTIVE COLORING

155. If all the proper care and thought is put into your hair color or lightening service, what may still cause problems that require color correction?

a) _____

b) _____

156. What can cause gray hair to have a yellow cast?

a) _____

b) _____

c) _____

d) _____

157. Which of the following should not be used to correct a yellow discoloration?

_____ a) lightener

_____ b) tint remover

_____ c) violet-based colors

_____ d) orange-based colors

158. Will hair color at a level nine or lighter give complete gray coverage? Why or why not?

_____

159. What result will be achieved by using a dark hair color on a salt-and-pepper head?

_____

160. _____ is the process of treating gray or very resistant hair to allow for better penetration of color.

161. Pre-softening is considered a:

_____ a) single- application hair coloring service

_____ b) double-application hair coloring service

_____ c) triple-application hair coloring service

_____ d) quadruple- application hair coloring service

162. List the guidelines to keep in mind when correcting color:

a) _____   e) _____

b) _____   f) _____

c) _____   g) _____

d) _____

163. Hair is considered damaged when it has one or more of the following characteristics:

a) _____   e) _____

b) _____   f) _____

c) _____   g) _____

d) _____

164. Prior to a tinting or lightening treatment, damaged hair should receive reconditioning treatments prior to and after the application of these chemical processes.

_____ True

_____ False

165. _____ are specialized preparations designed to help equalize porosity and deposit a base color in one application.

166. The two types of fillers are:

_____

167. _____ are used to recondition damaged, overly porous hair.

168. _____ are often demi-permanent color products that are used when there is doubt as to whether the color result will be an even shade.

169. List the advantages of using color fillers:

a) _____

b) _____

c) _____

d) _____

e) _____

f) _____

170. To obtain satisfactory results, select the color filler that will replace the _____ in your formulation.

171. Fading is a common problem with color-treated_____ hair.

    a) blonde

    b) red

    c) brown

    d) black

172. What causes fading?

_____

173. What should you consider when working with reds?

    a) _____

    _____

    b) _____

    _____

    c) _____

    _____

    d) _____

    _____

174. How should you camouflage excessive brassiness in tinted hair?

_____

_____

175. A prepared commercial product designed to remove artificial pigment from the hair is known

    as a_____.

176. How do tint removers work?

_____

_____

SALON MENU OF SERVICES

177. What is booking time?

_____

178. Describe each of the following services as you might find them in a salon's menu of services:

a) Single-process color/color enhancement: _____

_____

_____

b) Single-process retouch color with a glaze: _____

_____

_____

c) Double-process color: _____

_____

_____

d) Double-process retouch: _____

_____

_____

e) Dimensional hair color: _____

_____

_____

f) Special effects highlighting: _____

_____

_____

g) Corrective color: _____

_____

_____

17

HISTOLOGY OF THE SKIN

Date: _____

Rating:_____

Text Pages: 605-629

POINT TO PONDER:

"From the little spark may burst a mighty flame."—Dante

ANATOMY OF THE SKIN

1. The medical branch of science that deals with the study of skin and its nature, structure, functions,

    diseases, and treatment is called _____.

2. A _____ is a physician engaged in the science of treating the skin, its structures,

    functions, and diseases. An _____ is a specialist in the cleansing, preservation of health,

    and beautification of the skin and body.

3. Healthy skin is:

    a) _____

    b) _____

    c) _____

    d) _____

4. The appendages of the skin include:

    a) _____

    b) _____

    c) _____

    d) _____

5. The thinnest skin is on the palms and soles.

_____ True

_____ False

6. The skin is composed of two main divisions: the _____ and the _____.

7. The _____ is the outermost layer of the skin. This layer is also called the _____ or _____ and it forms a _____ for the body.

8. The epidermis is made up of the following layers:

a) _____

b) _____

c) _____

d) _____

9. The _____ is the underlying or inner layer of the skin.

10. Within the structure of the dermis, there are numerous:

a) _____   e) _____

b) _____   f) _____

c) _____   g) _____

d) _____

11. The dermis is made up of two layers called the _____ and the _____ _____.

12. Match the term with its correct description:

_____ 1. papillary layer   A. gives smoothness and contour to the body

_____ 2. dermal papillae   B. fatty layer found below the dermis

_____ 3. tactile corpuscles   C. outer layer of the dermis

_____ 4. subcutaneous tissue   D. nerve endings that are sensitive to touch and pressure

_____ 5. adipose tissue   E. small, cone-shaped elevations at the bottom of the hair follicles

13. The reticular layer contains the following structures within its network:

a) _____   e) _____

b) _____   f) _____

c) _____   g) _____

d) _____

14. Identify the parts of the skin illustrated below.

1. _____

2. _____

3. _____

4. _____

5. _____

6. _____

7. _____

8. _____

9. _____

10. _____

11. _____

12. _____

13. _____

14. _____

15. _____

16. _____

17. _____

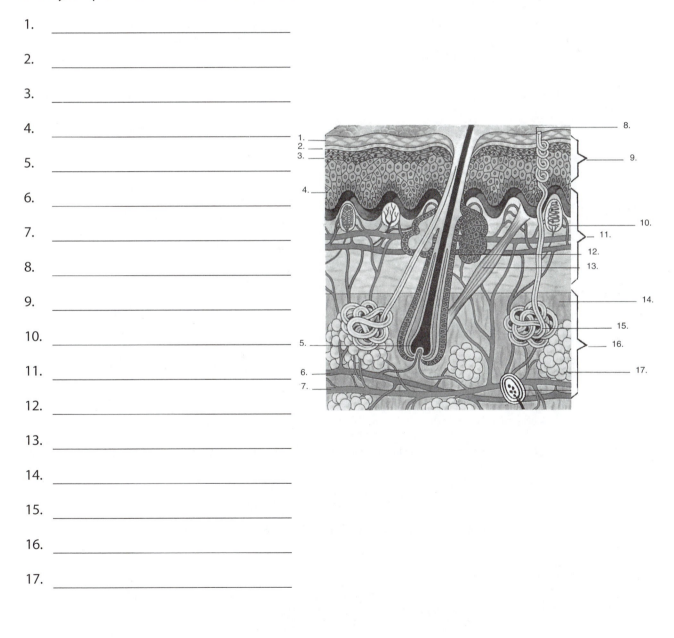

15. _____ , the clear fluids of the body that resemble blood plasma but contain only

colorless corpuscles, supply nourishment to the skin.

16. As they circulate through the skin, the blood and lymph contribute essential materials for:

_____ a) hair follicles to grow shiny hair

_____ b) growth, nourishment, and repair of the skin, hair, and nails

_____ c) growth of super hard finger and toe nails

_____ d) blemishes and blackheads

17. Match the following nerve fibers with their descriptions:

_____ 1. motor nerve fibers   A. regulate the excretion of perspiration and control sebum

_____ 2. sensory nerve fibers   B. cause goose bumps when a person is frightened or cold

_____ 3. secretory nerve fibers C. react to heat, cold, touch, pressure, and pain

18. Nerve endings are most abundant in the:

_____ a) nose

_____ b) ears

_____ c) fingertips

_____ d) elbows

19. The color of the skin depends primarily on _____ , the tiny grains of pigment deposited in the

stratum germinativum of the epidermis and the papillary layers of the dermis.

20. The acronym SPF stands for:

_____ a) skin peeling factor

_____ b) sarcoma pedis factor

_____ c) sun protection factor

_____ d) sun paralysis factor

21. The skin gets its strength, form, and flexibility from two specific structures composed of flexible protein

fibers found within the dermis called _____ and _____ .

22. _____ is a fibrous protein that gives the skin form and strength.

23. Collagen fibers are interwoven with _____ , a protein base similar to collagen that forms elastic

tissue. This fiber gives the skin its flexibility and elasticity.

24. What happens to collagen and elastin as we age?

_____

25. The skin contains two types of duct glands, _____ and

_____ , that extract materials from the blood to form new substances.

26. The sudoriferous glands excrete:

_____ a) oil

_____ b) fragrance

_____ c) sweat

_____ d) water

27. The sweat glands regulate _____ and help to eliminate _____

from the body.

28. The sebaceous or oil glands of the skin are connected to the _____ .

29. _____ is a fatty or oily secretion that lubricates the skin and preserves the softness of the hair.

30. Sebaceous glands are *not* found on the:

_____ a) scalp

_____ b) face

_____ c) palms

_____ d) knees

31. When sebum hardens and the sebaceous duct becomes clogged, a _____ is formed.

32. The principal functions of the skin are:

a) _____

b) _____

c) _____

d) _____

e) _____

f) _____

33. Name the factors that influence the aging of the skin.

   a) _____

   b) _____

   c) _____

   d) _____

34. Approximately what percentage of aging in skin is caused by the rays of the sun?

   _____ a) 60%-65%

   _____ b) 70%-75%

   _____ c) 80% to 85%

   _____ d) 90%-95%

35. _____ rays, also called the "aging rays," contribute to 90 to 95% of the sun's ultraviolet rays

   that reach the earth's surface.

36. UVB rays weaken the collagen and elastin fibers, causing wrinkling and sagging in the tissues.

   _____ True

   _____ False

37. _____ rays cause tanning of the skin by affecting the melanocytes.

38. List ways to protect the skin from the damage of UVA and UVB exposure:

   a) _____

   b) _____

   c) _____

   d) _____

   e) _____

   f) _____

39. If any changes in coloration, size, or shape of a mole are detected, you should:

_____ a) see an esthetician

_____ b) see a dermatologist

_____ c) see a cosmetologist

_____ d) see a make up technician

40. What is the best defense against pollutants?

_____

_____

_____

41. What affect does each of the following have on the skin?

smoking   _____

nicotine   _____

illegal drugs _____

alcohol   _____

DISORDERS OF THE SKIN

42. A _____ is an injury that changes the structure of tissues or organs.

43. Match each of the following primary lesions with its description:

_____ 1. bulla   A. small blister or sac containing clear fluid

_____ 2. cyst   B. swelling

_____ 3. macule   C. closed, abnormally developed sac, containing fluid, semi-fluid, or
                                morbid matter, above or below the skin

_____ 4. papule   D. large blister containing a watery fluid; similar to a vesicle but larger

_____ 5. pustule   E. itchy, swollen lesion that lasts only a few hours

_____ 6. tubercle   F. inflamed pimple containing pus

_____ 7. tumor   G. abnormal rounded, solid lump above, within, or under the skin

_____ 8. vesicle   H. pimple

_____ 9. wheal   I. spot or discoloration on the skin, such as a freckle

44. Identify the primary lesions illustrated below.

1. _____

2. _____

3. _____

4. _____

5. _____

6. _____

7. _____

8. _____

9. _____

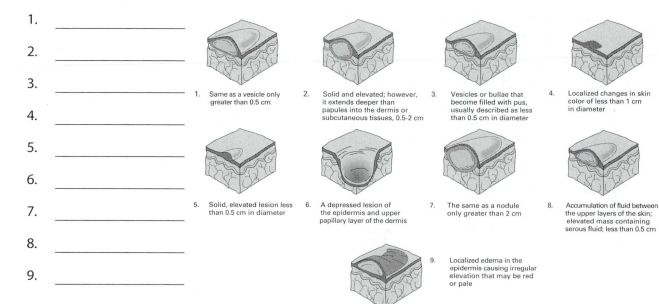

1. Same as a vesicle only greater than 0.5 cm

2. Solid and elevated; however, it extends deeper than papules into the dermis or subcutaneous tissues, 0.5-2 cm

3. Vesicles or bullae that become filled with pus, usually described as less than 0.5 cm in diameter

4. Localized changes in skin color of less than 1 cm in diameter

5. Solid, elevated lesion less than 0.5 cm in diameter

6. A depressed lesion of the epidermis and upper papillary layer of the dermis

7. The same as a nodule only greater than 2 cm

8. Accumulation of fluid between the upper layers of the skin; elevated mass containing serous fluid; less than 0.5 cm

9. Localized edema in the epidermis causing irregular elevation that may be red or pale

45. Match each of the following secondary lesions with its description:

_____ 1. crust

_____ 2. excoriation

_____ 3. fissure

_____ 4. keloid

_____ 5. scale

_____ 6. scar

_____ 7. ulcer

A. thick scar resulting from excessive growth of fibrous tissue

B. light-colored, slightly raised mark on the skin formed after a skin injury is healed

C. open lesion on the skin or mucous membrane of the body, accompanied by pus and loss of skin depth

D. dead cells that form over a wound or blemish while it is healing

E. skin sore or abrasion produced by scratching or scraping

F. crack in the skin that penetrates the dermis

G. any thin plate of epidermal flakes, dry or oily

46. Identify the secondary skin lesions as illustrated below.

1. _____

2. _____

3. _____

4. _____

5. _____

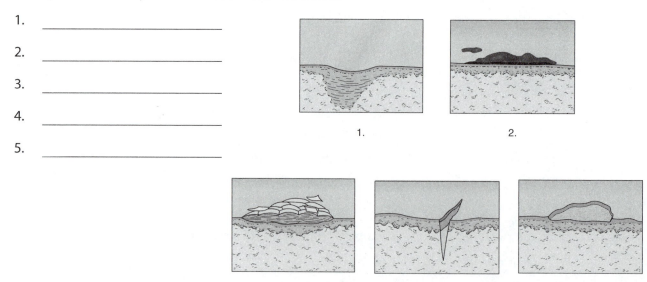

1.

2.

3.

4.

5.

47. Match each of the following disorders of the sebaceous glands with its description:

_____ 1. comedone

_____ 2. milia

_____ 3. acne

_____ 4. seborrhea

_____ 5. asteatosis

_____ 6. rosacea

_____ 7. steatoma

A. chronic congestion and dilation of the blood vessels

B. abnormal increase of secretion from the sebaceous glands

C. dry, scaly skin due to a deficiency or absence of sebum

D. sebaceous cyst or fatty tumor

E. small, whitish, pearlike masses in the epidermis due to retention of sebum

F. wormlike mass of hardened sebum in a hair follicle

G. chronic inflammation of the sebaceous glands from retained secretions

48. Match each of the following disorders of the sudoriferous glands with its description:

_____ 1. anhidrosis

_____ 2. bromhidrosis

_____ 3. hyperhidrosis

_____ 4. miliaria rubra

A. prickly heat

B. deficiency in perspiration

C. foul-smelling perspiration

D. excessive sweating

49. Match each of the following skin conditions with its description:

_____ 1. dermatitis

_____ 2. eczema

_____ 3. herpes simplex

_____ 4. psoriasis

A. inflammatory, painful itching disease of the skin

B. red patches covered with white-silver scales

C. inflammatory condition of the skin

D. fever blister or cold sore

50. Cosmetologists must be careful about skin disorders from frequent contact with chemicals such as

_____ .

51. Match each of the following skin pigmentations with its description:

_____ 1. albinism

_____ 2. chloasma

_____ 3. lentigines

_____ 4. leukoderma

_____ 5. nevus

_____ 6. stain

_____ 7. tan

_____ 8. vitiligo

A. change in pigmentation of skin caused by exposure to the sun or ultraviolet rays

B. freckles

C. abnormal brown or wine-colored skin discoloration

D. increased pigmentation on the skin, in spots that are not elevated

E. light abnormal patches

F. absence of melanin pigment of the body

G. milky-white spots

H. birthmark

52. A _____ of the skin is an abnormal growth of the skin.

53. Match the following with its description:

_____ 1. keratoma   A. Cutaneous outgrowth of the skin
_____ 2. mole   B. callus
_____ 3. skin tag   C. wart
_____ 4. verruca   D. small, brownish spot or blemish on the skin

54. _____ is the most common type of skin cancer and the least severe.

55. _____ is more serious than basal cell carcinoma and often is characterized by

scaly red papules or nodules.

56. The most serious form of skin cancer is _____ which is often characterized

by black or dark brown patches on the skin that may appear uneven in texture, jagged or raised.

MAINTAINING THE HEALTH OF THE SKIN

57. A major factor in maintaining the skin's overall health is _____.

58. Match the following vitamin with its effect on healthy skin:

_____ 1. vitamin A   A. promotes the healthy and rapid healing of the skin
_____ 2. vitamin C   B. aids in the health, function and repair of skin cells
_____ 3. vitamin D   C. helps fight against and protect the skin from sun damage
_____ 4. vitamin E   D. aids in and even speeds up the healing processes of the body

59. In its topical acid form, vitamin A is available as the prescription cream _____.

60. Drinking pure water is essential to the health of the skin and body because it:

a) _____

b) _____

c) _____

d) _____

18

HAIR REMOVAL

See Milady's Standard Cosmetology Practical Workbook

19

FACIALS

Date: _____

Rating: _____

Text Pages: 653-693

POINT TO PONDER:

"The wise person possesses humility. He knows that his small island of knowledge is surrounded by a vast sea of the unknown."—Harold C. Chase

BASIC CLASSIFICATION AND CHEMISTRY OF SKIN CARE PRODUCTS

1. The five main categories of skin care products are:

   a) _____   d) _____

   b) _____   e) _____

   c) _____

2. _____ are designed for every skin type and skin condition and come in three basic forms:

   face wash, cleansing lotion, and cleansing cream.

3. Match the following terms with their descriptions:

   _____ 1. Face wash   A. light-textured, oil-based emulsion used to dissolve makeup quickly.
   _____ 2. Cleansing lotion   B. agents that soften or smooth the skin surface.
   _____ 3. Emollients   C. detergent-type foaming cleanser with a neutral or slightly acidic pH
   _____ 4. Cleansing cream   D. water-based emulsion, used twice a day on normal and combination
                                  skin

4. Fresheners, toners (or tonics), and _____ all perform three specific functions:

   a) _____

   b) _____

   c) _____

   _____

5. Match each of the following tonic lotions with its strength and alcohol content:

    _____ 1. Fresheners   A. up to 35% alcohol content

    _____ 2. Toners (or tonics) B. 0 to 4% alcohol content

    _____ 3. Astringents   C. 4 to 15% alcohol content

6. Tonic lotions can be applied to the face _____ or they can be _____

    _____ .

7. The term "exfoliation" refers to the peeling and shredding of the horny layer of the skin.

    _____ True

    _____ False

8. A/an _____ is an ingredient that assists in the process of exfoliating the skin.

9. During the process of _____ , some method of physical contact is used to

    literally scrape or bump cells off the skin.

10. The removal of dry, dead surface cells can help the skin in the following ways:

     a) _____

     b) _____

     c) _____

     d) _____

     e) _____

     f) _____

11. You should not use brushing machines, scrubs, or any harsh mechanical peeling techniques on these
     skin types and conditions:

     a) _____

     b) _____

     c) _____

     d) _____

     _____

     _____

     e) _____

12. Describe what occurs during microdermabrasion:

_____

_____

13. A chemical exfoliation is also known as an _____ and involves the use of

substances called _____, which help speed up the breakdown of keratin,

the protein in skin.

14. What is a vegetal peeling or a gommage?

_____

_____

_____

15. How is a powdered form of enzyme peel used?

_____

_____

_____

16. Enzyme peelings are suitable for the following conditions:

   a) _____

   _____

   b) _____

   _____

   c) _____

   _____

   d) _____

   _____

17. Alphahydroxy acids are derived from:

_____

18. How do alphahydroxy acids work?

   _____

   _____

   _____

19. Alphahydroxy acid exfoliation may be administered anytime to any client.

   _____ True

   _____ False

20. _____ , are designed to hydrate and condition the skin during the night, when normal tissue repair is taking place.

21. _____ are lubricants with very little or no active ingredients and are designed to give the practitioner a good slip during massage, so that the skin is not stretched.

22. _____ are products formulated to add moisture to dry skin; they are water-based emulsions, which are absorbed quickly without leaving any residue on the surface of the skin.

23. A valuable ingredient found in a moisturizer is _____ ; which helps guard against premature aging of the skin, and, when used consistently, is one of the best ways to help prevent skin cancer.

24. _____ are special cosmetic preparations applied to the face to benefit and beautify the skin; they require a short application time and allow a practitioner to treat different skin conditions on the same face at the same time.

25. A _____ is usually a setting product, which means that it dries after application and provides a complete closure to the environment on top of the skin.

26. Masks use the following special ingredients to achieve their tightening and sebum-absorbing effects:

    a) _____

    b) _____

    c) _____

27. _____ are ready-to-use masks used to stimulate circulation and

    temporarily contract the pores of the skin.

28. _____ are specially prepared facial masks containing paraffin and other

    beneficial ingredients that are melted at a little more than body temperature before application.

29. _____ contain special crystals of gypsum, a plaster-like ingredient.

30. The chemical reaction that occurs when the plaster and the crystals of the modelage mask mix with
    water produces a gradually increasing temperature that reaches approximately:

    _____ a) 96 degrees Fahrenheit

    _____ b) 99 degrees Fahrenheit

    _____ c) 102 degrees Fahrenheit

    _____ d) 105 degrees Fahrenheit

31. _____ contain a common chemical as their most important ingredient

    and have been found to have a beneficial effect in reducing the production of sebum.

32. _____ , also referred to as cream masks or gel masks, are very similar in

    composition to treatment creams in that they remain soft and creamy throughout their entire setting

    time.

33. _____ are small, sealed glass vials containing a single application of a

    highly concentrated extract in a water or oil base.

CLIENT CONSULTATION

34. All facial treatments should begin with a thorough _____ .

35. The record card should contain the following information:

   a) _____
   _____

   b) _____
   _____

   c) _____
   _____

   d) _____
   _____

   e) _____
   _____

   f) _____
   _____

   g) _____
   _____

   h) _____
   _____

   i) _____
   _____

36. As part of the consultation, do not hesitate to:

   a) _____

   b) _____

   c) _____

37. Match the following skin types with their descriptions:

    _____ 1. oily skin   A. may have either oily and normal areas or normal and dry areas

    _____ 2. normal skin   B. lacking in oil; often dehydrated

    _____ 3. dry skin   C. has overabundance of sebum; may or may not be blemished

    _____ 4. combination skin   D. usually in good condition; has adequate supply of sebum and moisture

38. If oily skin is not cleansed properly, sebum and dead cells can clog pores and lead to _____.

39. _____ can occur in all skin types as a reaction to such enemies of the skin as air pollution, chemicals present in water, and preservatives in food.

40. _____ can occur in every skin type, regardless of how oily the skin is, because of an insufficient amount of water in the body.

41. On your consultation card you should include any skin abnormalities you observe, such as abnormalities of:

    a) _____

    b) _____

    c) _____

    d) _____

    e) _____

    f) _____

FACIAL MASSAGE

42. _____ is the manual or mechanical manipulation of the body by rubbing, pinching, kneading, tapping, and other movements to increase metabolism and circulation, promote absorption, and relieve pain.

43. To master massage techniques, you must have a basic knowledge of _____ and _____ as well as considerable practice in performing the various movements.

44. To prepare to give massage. you should:

    a) _____

    _____

    b) _____

    _____

    c) _____

    _____

    d) _____

    _____

45. Every muscle has a _____ , which is a point on the skin over the muscle where

    pressure or stimulation will cause contraction of that muscle.

46. Identify the motor nerve points on the illustration below.

    1. _____

    2. _____

    3. _____

    4. _____

    5. _____

    6. _____

47. Relaxation is achieved through _____ or

    _____ .

48. The following benefits may be obtained by proper facial and scalp massage:

    a) _____

    b) _____

    c) _____

    d) _____

    e) _____

    f) _____

    g) _____

ELECTROTHERAPY AND LIGHT THERAPY

49. Electrical facial treatments are called _____.

50. The currents used in electrical facial and scalp treatments are referred to as _____.

51. The modalities that concern cosmetologists are: _____

_____ currents.

52. An_____ is an applicator for directing the electric current from the machine to the client's skin.

53. A negative electrode is called a _____, has a black plug and cord, and is marked with an "N" or a minus (-) sign.

54. A positive electrode is called an_____, has a red plug and cord, and is marked with a "P" or a plus (+) sign.

55. The most commonly used electrotherapy device is the _____ which produces significant chemical changes.

56. How will your client experience the effects of the galvanic current?

_____

57. The_____ electrode is the electrode used on the area to be treated and the _____ electrode will be held by your client in some fashion in order for the circuit to be completed.

58. _____ refers to the application of light rays to the skin for the treatment of disorders.

59. Match the type of light listed below with its effect on the skin:

_____ 1. ultraviolet   A. improves dry, scaly, wrinkled skin
_____ 2. infrared   B. relieves pain in the back of the neck and shoulders.
_____ 3. white Light   C. soothes nerves
_____ 4. blue Light   D. heats and relaxes the skin.
_____ 5. red Light   E. increases the elimination of waste products.

60. Artificial light rays are produced by an electrical apparatus called a _____.

FACIAL TREATMENTS

61. Facial treatments fall under two categories:

a) _____   b) _____

62. Facial treatments help to:

a) _____   d) _____

b) _____   e) _____

c) _____

63. After the client is draped and seated in the facial chair, you should inspect the skin to:

a) _____   d) _____

_____   _____

b) _____   e) _____

_____   _____

c) _____   f) _____

_____   _____

64. The results of your analysis will determine:

a) _____

b) _____

c) _____

d) _____

65. _____ is the process of softening and emulsifying grease deposits and

blackheads in the follicles for easier extraction.

66. What is the process of iontophoresis used for?

_____

_____

_____

67. What are faradic and sinusoidal currents used for?

_____

_____

_____

68. What is the high-frequency current used for?

_____

_____

_____

69. Pack facials are recommended for which skin type?

_____ a) dry skin only

_____ b) oily skin only

_____ c) aging skin only

_____ d) all skin types

70. Masks are recommended for:

_____ a) combination skin

_____ b) oily skin

_____ c) dry and mature skin

_____ d) blemished skin

AROMATHERAPY

71. The therapeutic use of essential oils is called _____.

72. The skilled use of essential oils can enhance a person's _____

_____.

20

FACIAL MAKEUP

Date: _____

Rating:_____

Text Pages: 695-734

POINT TO PONDER:

"To love oneself is the beginning of a lifelong romance."—Oscar Wilde

1. The main objective of facial makeup is to _____

   _____ .

2. When applying makeup you must take into consideration the:

   a) _____   d) _____

   b) _____   e) _____

   c) _____

3. You can use makeup to create optical illusions with _____ .

COSMETICS FOR FACIAL MAKEUP

4. _____ is a cosmetic, usually tinted, that is used as a base or as a protective film

   applied before makeup and/or powder.

5. Foundation is used to:

   a) _____

   b) _____

   c) _____

6. List the most widely used types of foundation:

   a) _____   c) _____

   b) _____   d) _____

7. _____ are predominantly water, mineral oil, stearic acid, cetyl alcohol, propylene glycol, triethanolamine, lanolin derivatives, borax, and insoluble pigments and are generally suited for dry to normal skin and give medium to full coverage.

8. _____ are suspensions of organic and inorganic pigments in alcohol and water-based solutions and are generally suited for clients with oily to normal skin conditions that desire a sheer to medium coverage foundation.

9. _____ consist of a powder base mixed with a coloring agent (pigment) and perfume, and are especially effective for oily skin.

10. _____ are moist on application but dry to a powdery finish.

11. Why is foundation so important to the entire makeup application?

_____

12. Skin tones are generally classified as: _____ , _____ , or _____ .

13. Match each of the following skin tones to the colors it describes:

_____ 1. Warm tones   A. blue, blue-green, or blue-red

_____ 2. Cool tones   B. equal amounts of warm and cool tones

_____ 3. Neutral   C. yellow, orange, or red-orange

14. Foundation should always be one shade darker than the person's actual skin tone.

_____ True
_____ False

15. The best way to determine the correct foundation color for your client is to apply a stripe of color to clean skin on the:

_____ a) elbow
_____ b) palm
_____ c) jawline
_____ d) forearm

16. You will know you have the correct foundation color if after blending slightly the color:

    _____ a) looks slightly pink

    _____ b) looks slightly yellow

    _____ c) glows

    _____ d) disappears

17. _____ are used to cover blemishes and discolorations and may be

    applied before or after foundation.

18. Match the type of concealer listed below with the type of coverage it provides:

    _____ 1. pot concealer   A. provides sheer to medium coverage.
    _____ 2. pencil concealer   B. provides medium to sheer coverage.
    _____ 3. wand concealer   C. provides the most coverage.

19. Concealer is used sparingly over _____ or _____ and

    blended into the surrounding skin with a facial sponge.

20. You will know you have the correct color of concealer if, after applying it, the color:

    _____ a) looks slightly pink

    _____ b) llooks slightly yellow

    _____ c) glows

    _____ d) matches the skin

21. _____ is a fine cosmetic powder, sometimes tinted and scented, that

    is used to add a matte or dull finish to the face.

22. Face powder increases the overall attractiveness of the skin by:

    a) _____

    b) _____

    c) _____

23. Face powder consists of a _____ base mixed with a _____

    and perfume.

24. Ingredients in most powders include: _____

_____.

25. Face powder is applied:

_____ a) before foundation

_____ b) before concealer

_____ c) after foundation

_____ d) after blush

26. _____, also called blush, blusher, or rouge, is a cream or powder

cosmetic used to color the cheeks and the skin beneath the cheekbones.

27. Blush should give a _____ to the face and also helps to create more

attractive facial contours.

28. Powder cheek color is simply compact or pressed powder with _____ added.

29. Cream cheek colors fall into two categories: _____ and _____.

30. _____ is a cosmetic in paste form, usually in a metal or plastic tube,

manufactured in a variety of colors and used to color the lips and enhance or correct the shape of the lips.

31. Lip color is available in a variety of forms: _____, _____ ,_____,

_____ , and_____.

32. All lip color formulas include:_____, _____,

and_____.

33. _____ is a colored pencil used to outline the lips and help to keep lip

color from feathering.

34. When is lip liner usually applied?

_____

35. _____ are a cosmetic applied on the eyelids to accentuate or

    contour them.

36. Eye shadow is available in _____ and _____ form.

37. When applied to the lids, eye color or shadow makes the eyes appear_____ and

    _____ .

38. When applying eye shadow, you should match eye shadow to eye color.

    _____ True

    _____ False

39. A darker shade of eye shadow makes the natural color of the iris appear_____ , while

    a lighter shade makes the iris appear _____ .

40. Eye colors and shadows are available in_____ , _____ , _____ ,

    and_____ form, and usually come with an applicator.

41. Match each of the following eye shadows with its description:

    _____ 1. Highlight color   A. A medium tone used to even skin tone on the eye.

    _____ 2. Base color   B. A deep shade used to minimize a specific area.

    _____ 3. Contour color   C. A shade lighter than the client's skin tone used to make an area
                                         appear larger.

42. _____ is a cosmetic used to outline and emphasize the eyes.

43. Eyeliner is used to _____

    _____ .

44. Eyeliner pencils consist of a _____ or hardened _____ with a

    variety of additives to create color.

45. _____ are used to add color and shape to the eyebrows, usually after tweezing or waxing.

46. _____ is a cosmetic preparation used to darken, define, and thicken the eyelashes.

47. Mascara is available in _____ , _____ , and _____ form and a variety of shades and tints.

48. Mascara is available in _____ and _____ .

49. _____ remove eye makeup products that are water-resistant.

50. _____ is a heavy makeup used for theatrical purposes.

51. List the most commonly used makeup brushes:

a) _____   e) _____

b) _____   f) _____

c) _____   g) _____

d) _____   h) _____

52. Disposable implements important to the makeup artist include:

a) _____   f) _____

b) _____   g) _____

c) _____   h) _____

d) _____   i) _____

e) _____

MAKEUP COLOR THEORY

53. Match the following terms with their descriptions:

     _____ 1. primary colors   A. formed by mixing equal amounts of a secondary color and its neighboring primary color on the color wheel

     _____ 2. secondary colors   B. fundamental colors that cannot be obtained from a mixture

     _____ 3. tertiary colors   C. obtained by mixing equal parts of two primary colors

54. The primary colors are _____ , _____ , and _____ .

55. A primary and secondary color directly opposite each other on the color wheel are called

_____ .

56. When mixed, complementary colors cancel each other out to create a _____

color.

57. When complementary colors are placed next to each other, each color makes the other look

_____ , resulting in greater contrast.

58. _____ are the range of colors from yellow and gold through oranges,

red-oranges, most reds, and some yellow-greens.

59. _____ are dominated by blues, greens, violets and blue-reds.

60. Red is a warm color.

     _____ True

     _____ False

61. There are three main factors to consider when choosing colors for a client: _____ ,

_____ , and _____ .

62. When determining skin color, you must first decide if the skin is _____ , _____ ,

or _____ in level, and then you must determine whether the tone of the skin is _____

or _____ .

63. Fill in the correct tone for each category below:

Skin Color	Warm	Cool
light skin		
medium skin		
dark skin		

64. A _____ skin tone contains equal elements of warm and cool, no matter

how light or dark the skin is.

CLIENT CONSULTATION

65. Describe the type of lighting that is required for a makeup consultation area:

_____

_____

_____

66. What information should you record on the consultation card?

a) _____

b) _____

c) _____

d) _____

e) _____

f) _____

67. What is special occasion makeup?

_____

CORRECTIVE MAKEUP

68. Corrective makeup techniques are used to _____
    _____.

69. Determining a person's face shape allows you to _____
    _____.

21

NAIL STRUCTURE AND GROWTH

Date: _____

Rating:_____

Text Pages: 737-755

POINT TO PONDER:

"Thought, not money, is the real business capital, and if you know absolutely that what you are doing is right, then you are bound to accomplish it in due season."—Harvey Firestone

THE NAIL

1. The_____ is the horny protective plate located at the end of the finger or toe.

2. The nail is an appendage of the skin and is therefore part of the:

    _____ a) respiratory system

    _____ b) integumentary system

    _____ c) circulatory system

    _____ d) skeletal system

3. A normal, healthy nail is firm and flexible and should be shiny and slightly_____ in color.

4. The nail is composed mainly of _____ , the same protein found in skin and hair, and is

    technically referred to as:

    _____ a) ruby

    _____ b) onyx

    _____ c) pearl

    _____ d) diamond

5. The nail is quite _____ ; water will pass through it much more easily than it will pass

    through normal skin.

6. The nail unit consists of six basic parts:

   a) _____   d) _____

   b) _____   e) _____

   c) _____   f) _____

7. The nail anatomy is the same in both fingernails and toenails.

   _____ True

   _____ False

8. The _____ is the portion of the skin upon which the nail plate rests and because it is supplied with blood vessels, it is seen as a pinkish area extending from the lunula to the area just before the free edge of the nail.

9. The nail bed is supplied with many nerves and is attached to the nail plate by a thin layer of tissue called the _____.

10. The _____ is where the nail is formed and is composed of matrix cells that produce the nail plate.

11. The visible portion of the matrix bed is called the _____.

12. The horny _____ rests on and is attached to the nail bed.

13. The _____ is the part of the nail plate that extends over the tip of the finger or toe.

14. The _____ is the crescent of toughened skin around the base of the fingernails and toenails.

15. The _____ is the extension of the cuticle at the base of the nail body that partly overlaps the lunula.

16. The _____ is the thickened stratum corneum of the epidermis that lies underneath the free edge of the nail.

17. A _____ is a tough band of fibrous tissue that connects bones or holds an organ

in place.

18. The_____ are folds of normal skin that surround the nail plate.

19. What do nail folds form?

_____

20. The deep fold of skin in which the matrix bed is lodged is called the _____.

21. Identify the parts of the nail as illustrated below.

1. _____

2. _____

3. _____

4. _____

5. _____

6. _____

7. _____

8. _____

9. _____

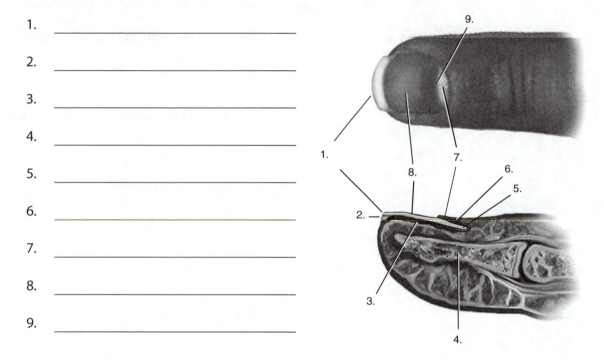

NAIL GROWTH

22. The factors that affect nail growth are _____ and _____.

23. A normal nail grows:

_____ a) forward, starting at the free edge and extending over the tip of the finger.

_____ b) forward, starting at the matrix and extending over the tip of the finger.

_____ c) backward starting at the free edge and extending back towards the half moon.

_____ d) Backward stating at the lanula and extending back over the eponychium.

24. The average rate of nail growth in the normal adult is about:

    _____ a) ½" per month

    _____ b) ½" per week

    _____ c) ⅛" per month

    _____ d) ⅛" per week

25. Malformation of the nail is caused by _____ , _____ ,

    or_____

26. A _____ is a condition caused by injury to the nail or some disease or imbalance

    in the body.

27. You can help your clients with nail disorders by:

    a) _____

    _____

    b) _____

    _____

28. Match each of the following nail disorders with its description:

    _____ 1. blue nails   A. when the edges of the nail plate curl around at the free edge
    _____ 2. bruised nails   B. folded nail
    _____ 3. corrugations   C. usually the result of illness or from an injury to the nail cells in the matrix
    _____ 4. eggshell nails   D. overgrowth of the nail, usually in thickness rather than length
    _____ 5. furrows   E. abnormal brittleness with striation of the nail plate
    _____ 6. hangnail   F. bitten nails
    _____ 7. infected finger   G. atrophy or wasting away of the nail
    _____ 8. leukonychia   H. darkening of the fingernails or toenails
    _____ 9. melanonychia   I. forward growth of the eponychium with adherence to the nail surface
    _____ 10. onychatrophia   J. when the cuticle splits around the nail
    _____ 11. onychauxis   K. creased crosswise curvature throughout the nail plate
    _____ 12. onychophagy   L. finger is red, painful, swollen or filled with pus
    _____ 13. onychorrhexis   M. whitish discoloration of the nails, caused by injury to the base of the nail
    _____ 14. plicatured nail   N. noticeably thin, white nail plate, are more flexible than normal
    _____ 15. pterygium   O. a blood clot forms under the nail plate, forming a dark purplish spot
    _____ 16. tile-shaped nails   P. uneven growth of the nails, usually the result of illness or injury
    _____ 17. trumpet nail   Q. poor blood circulation, a heart disorder, or topical and oral medications

NAIL FUNGUS

29. _____ are vegetable parasites, including all types of fungus and mold, and

    usually appear under the nails of the hands and feet as a _____ , _____

    residue that progresses to a _____ and _____ texture under the nail plate.

30. Discolorations between the nail plate and artificial enhancements are a bacterial infection caused by

    bacteria called _____ .

31. Infection results from _____

    _____ .

NAIL DISEASES

32. Match each of the following nail diseases with its description:

    _____ 1. onychosis   A. a vegetable parasite, or fungus
    _____ 2. onychia   B. ingrown nails
    _____ 3. onychocryptosis   C. any deformity or disease of the nails
    _____ 4. onychogryposis   D. ringworm of the nails
    _____ 5. onycholysis   E. periodic shedding of one or more nails, in whole or in part
    _____ 6. onychomadesis   F. severe inflammation in which a lump of red tissue grows up from
                                          the nail bed to the nail plate
    _____ 7. onychophosis   G. thickening and increased curvature of the nail
    _____ 8. onychoptosis   H. separation and falling off of a nail from the nail bed
    _____ 9. paronychia   I. loosening of the nail without shedding
    _____ 10. pyogenic granuloma   J. bacterial inflammation of the tissues surrounding the nail
    _____ 11. tinea   K. athlete's foot
    _____ 12. tinea pedis   L. inflammation of the nail matrix, including pus and shedding of
                                          the nail
    _____ 13. tinea unguium   M. growth of horny epithelium in the nail bed

22

MANICURING AND PEDICURING

See Milady's Standard Cosmetology Practical Workbook

23

ADVANCED NAIL TECHNIQUES

See Milady's Standard Cosmetology Practical Workbook

24

THE SALON BUSINESS

Date: _____

Rating:_____

Text Pages: 827-853

POINT TO PONDER:

"It is better to have a permanent income than to be fascinating."—Oscar Wilde

GOING INTO BUSINESS FOR YOURSELF

1. The two main options for becoming your own boss are _____

_____.

2. Describe a booth rental arrangement.

_____

_____

3. Does a booth renter have any obligation to the salon owner?

_____

4. What are the advantages of booth renting?

_____

_____

5. What are the obligations a booth renter must assume?

_____

6. When you consider opening a salon you should read and research the following extensively:

_____

_____

7. List the elements of a good business location:

a) _____

b) _____

c) _____

d) _____

e) _____

8. What is meant by an area's demographics?

_____

9. How should you determine whether or not another salon in your area is a direct competitor to your salon?

_____

_____

10. Which of the following best describes a business plan?

_____ a) a wish list

_____ b) a profit and loss statement

_____ c) a map

_____ d) a job description

11. What should be included in your business plan?

a) _____

_____

b) _____

_____

c) _____

_____

d) _____

_____

e) _____

_____

12. What kind of laws must be complied with when you open a salon?

_____

13. What kind of insurance must be purchased when you open your business?

a) _____

b) _____

c) _____

d) _____

14. What are the three types of salon ownership?

a) _____

b) _____

c) _____

15. Describe a business that is owned by a sole proprietor.

_____

_____

16. Describe a partnership.

_____

_____

_____

17. Describe a business owned by a corporation.

_____

_____

_____

18. If you choose to buy an established salon, your agreement should include the following:

a) _____

_____

b) _____

_____

c) _____

_____

d) _____

_____

e) _____

_____

f) _____

_____

g) _____

_____

19. In many cases, owning your own business does not mean that you own the building that houses your business.

_____ True

_____ False

20. A lease should specify the following:

a) _____

b) _____

c) _____

d) _____

21. What can you do to protect the salon against fire, theft, and lawsuits?

a) _____

b) _____

c) _____

d) _____

e) _____

22. Smooth business management depends on the following factors:

a) _____

b) _____

c) _____

d) _____

e) _____

f) _____

23. Match the following expense items with the figure that is a reasonable percentage of revenue to be spent on each:

_____ 1. salaries and commissions (including payroll taxes)   A. 1.0

_____ 2. rent   B. 53.5

_____ 3. supplies   C. 1.0

_____ 4. advertising   D. 1.5

_____ 5. depreciation   E. 5.0

_____ 6. laundry   F. 1.5

_____ 7. cleaning   G. 1.0

_____ 8. light and power   H. 3.0

_____ 9. repairs   I. 3.0

_____ 10. insurance   J. .75

_____ 11. telephone   K. 15.0

_____ 12. miscellaneous   L. 13.0

_____ 13. net profit   M. .75

24. Good business operation requires a simple and efficient record system.

_____ True

_____ False

25. What is your business's income derived from?

_____

26. List the types of expenses a salon may incur.

_____

27. Why is it important to record all business transactions?

a) _____

_____

b) _____

_____

c) _____

_____

d) _____

_____

28. Why should you keep financial records on a weekly or monthly basis?

    a) _____

    b) _____

    c) _____

    d) _____

29. Why should you keep daily records?

    a) _____

    _____

    b) _____

    _____

30. Purchase records help maintain a perpetual _____ , which prevents _____

    _____ of needed supplies, and can also alert you to any incidents of _____ .

31. Unscramble these words and use them to fill in the blanks below.

    ntisumcopon   tareil

    Supplies to be used in the daily business operation are _____ supplies. Those to be

    sold to clients are _____ supplies.

32. Service records should include:

    a) _____

    b) _____

    c) _____

    d) _____

    e) _____

    f) _____

OPERATING A SUCCESSFUL SALON

33. How can you ensure that you will stay in business and have a prosperous salon?

   _____

34. When planning the salon's layout, maximum _____ should be the primary concern.

35. List the things to be aware of to insure maximum efficiency:

   a) _____

   _____

   b) _____

   _____

   c) _____

   _____

   d) _____

   _____

   e) _____

   _____

   f) _____

   _____

   g) _____

   _____

   h) _____

   _____

   i) _____

   _____

   j) _____

   _____

   k) _____

   _____

36. What will determine the number of salon employees?

    _____

37. When interviewing potential employees, consider their: _____

    _____

38. What are some ways you can share your success with your staff:

    a) _____

    b) _____

    c) _____

    d) _____

    e) _____

    f) _____

    _____

    g) _____

39. What are the traits of an effective manager?

    a) _____

    b) _____

    c) _____

    d) _____

    e) _____

    f) _____

    g) _____

40. The best salons employ professional _____ to handle the job of scheduling

    appointments and greeting clients.

41. The reception area should be: _____.

42. The receptionist handles important functions such as: _____

    _____.

    _____.

43. The person who makes appointments and who answers the phone or deals with clients must have:

_____

_____ .

44. The telephone is used to:

a) _____

b) _____

c) _____

d) _____

e) _____

f) _____

g) _____

h) _____

45. When using the telephone, you should:

a) _____

b) _____

c) _____

d) _____

e) _____

46. When booking appointments, you should be familiar with _____

_____ .

47. If a client calls to make an appointment with a particular cosmetologist who is not available for the day or time the client requests, you should:

a) _____

b) _____

c) _____

48. How should customer complaints over the phone be handled?

a) _____

_____

b) _____

c) _____

d) _____

e) _____

f) _____

g) _____

49. What is advertising?

_____

_____

50. What does advertising do?

_____

_____

51. What forms of advertising are most useful to the salon?

a) _____   f) _____

b) _____   g) _____

c) _____   h) _____

d) _____   i) _____

e) _____   j) _____

SELLING IN THE SALON

52. An important aspect of the salon's financial success revolves around the sale of

_____ and _____ .

53. How should you and your staff view selling in the salon?

_____

_____

54. How should a stylist approach selling to clients?

_____

_____

25

SEEKING EMPLOYMENT

Date: _____

Rating: _____

Text Pages: 855-887

POINT TO PONDER:

"Action without study is fatal. Study without action is futile."—Mary Beard

PREPARING FOR LICENSURE

1. Being _____ means having a complete and thorough knowledge of your subject matter

   and understanding the strategies for taking tests successfully.

2. List the daily habits and time management skills of effective studying:

   a) _____

   b) _____

   c) _____

   d) _____

   e) _____

   f) _____

   g) _____

   h) _____

3. What holistic steps can you take to prepare for test-taking?

   a) _____

   b) _____

   c) _____

   d) _____

   e) _____

   f) _____

   g) _____

4. On the day of the exam you should begin quickly and read the directions for completing each section as you go.

_____ True

_____ False

5. It is okay to ask the test examiner questions if there is anything you do not understand.

_____ True

_____ False

6. Skim the entire test before beginning and answer the easiest questions first in order to save time for the more difficult ones.

_____ True

_____ False.

7. _____ is the process of reaching logical conclusions by employing logical reasoning.

8. When taking a test, you should begin by eliminating options that you know are incorrect.

_____ True

_____ False

9. In a true/false statement only part of the statement needs to be true.

_____ True

_____ False

10. When answering multiple-choice questions it is wise to eliminate completely incorrect answers first.

_____ True

_____ False

11. When answering matching questions it is best to read all items in each list before beginning.

_____ True

_____ False

12. When answering essay questions, make sure that what you write is _____,

    _____, _____, _____,

    and _____ .

13. In order to be successful at test-taking, you must follow the rules of_____ and

    be _____ for both the written

    and the practical examination.

14. In order to be better prepared for the practical portion of the examination, the new graduate should fol-
    low these tips:

    a) _____

    _____

    b) _____

    _____

    c) _____

    _____

    d) _____

    _____

    e) _____

    _____

    f) _____

    _____

    g) _____

    _____

    h) _____

    _____

    i) _____

    _____

PREPARING FOR EMPLOYMENT

15. List the key personal characteristics that will help you get and keep the position you want:

   a) _____

   b) _____

   c) _____

   d) _____

   e) _____

16. Match the following type of salon with the phrase that best describes it:

   _____ 1. small independent salons

   _____ 2. independent salon chains

   _____ 3. large national salon chains

   _____ 4. franchise salons

   A. salon chains that sell the right to use their name to individual owners

   B. management and marketing professionals at corporate headquarters make all the decisions for each salon

   C. usually owned by an individual, has one to three styling chairs

   D. ten or fewer salons owned by one individual or partners

17. Match the following type of salon with the phrase that best describes it:

   _____ 1. value-priced salon

   _____ 2. full-service salons

   _____ 3. image salons

   A. salons that offer luxurious, higher-priced services and treatments

   B. salons that depend on a high volume of traffic and charge low prices

   C. salons that offer a complete menu of hair, nail, and skin services

18. A _____ is a written summary of your education and work experience. It tells potential employers at a glance what your achievements and accomplishments are.

19. When preparing your professional resume you should:

   a) _____

   _____

   b) _____

   _____

   c) _____

   _____

d) _____

_____

e) _____

_____

f) _____

_____

g) _____

_____

20. An _____ is a collection, usually bound, of photos and documents

that reflect your skills, accomplishments, and abilities in your chosen career field.

21. A powerful employment portfolio includes:

a) _____

b) _____

c) _____

d) _____

e) _____

f) _____

g) _____

h) _____

i) _____

j) _____

22. List the points to consider when narrowing your job search for the best possible results:

a) _____

b) _____

c) _____

d) _____

e) _____

23. _____ allows you to establish contacts that may eventually lead to a job and that also help you gain valuable information about the workings of various establishments.

24. List the guidelines to follow when networking with local salons:

    a) _____

    _____

    b) _____

    _____

    c) _____

    _____

    d) _____

    _____

    e) _____

    _____

    f) _____

    _____

25. When you decide to make contact with an appropriate salon to ask for an interview you should send your resume only.

    _____ True

    _____ False

26. When getting ready for an interview, what five things should you be prepared for?

    a) _____

    b) _____

    c) _____

    d) _____

    e) _____

27. What behaviors should you practice in connection with the interview?

a) _____

b) _____

c) _____

d) _____

e) _____

f) _____

g) _____

h) _____

i) _____

j) _____

k) _____

l) _____

28. List some questions that you might consider asking during a job interview:

a) _____

b) _____

c) _____

d) _____

e) _____

f) _____

g) _____

h) _____

i) _____

j) _____

k) _____

29. Next to each question, indicate whether it is legal or illegal to be asked it in an interview:

How old are you?

Would you describe your medical history?

Are you over the age of 18?

Are you able to perform this job?

Are you a U.S. citizen?

Are you authorized to work in the U.S.?

In which languages are you fluent?

_____

_____

_____

_____

_____

_____

_____

YOU ARE ON YOUR WAY

30. List the best ways to use down time:

a) _____

b) _____

c) _____

d) _____

31. In order to remain healthy and energetic for your job you should:

a) _____

b) _____

c) _____

d) _____

e) _____

32. What should you do if you find yourself on a team with coworkers who bicker and gossip?

_____

DISCUSSION QUESTIONS

Answer the questions below and be prepared to discuss them in class at the appropriate time.

33. Why have you chosen a career in cosmetology?

_____

34. What do you really want out of a career in cosmetology?

_____

35. What particular areas within the beauty industry do you wish to concentrate on?

_____

36. What are your strongest practical skills and in what ways do you wish to use them?

_____

37. What personal qualities will help you have a successful career?

_____

26

ON THE JOB

Date: _____

Rating: _____

Text Pages: 889-910

POINT TO PONDER:

"When you do the common things in life in an uncommon way, you will command the attention of the world." - George Washington Carver

MOVING FROM SCHOOL TO WORK

1. Once you become the employee of a salon, you will be expected to put the needs of the _____

   _____ ahead of your own.

2. Putting the salon and clients' needs first means that you must always_____

   _____ and _____.

3. In order to be successful on the job, you need to find a salon that _____

   and_____.

4. Before considering a new job ask yourself the following questions:

   a) _____

   b) _____

   c) _____

   d) _____

OUT IN THE REAL WORLD

5. Many famous stylists began their careers as:

    _____ a) managers

    _____ b) estheticians

    _____ c) assistants

    _____ d) chemical specialists

6. Another entry-level salon job is:

    _____ a) color manager

    _____ b) perm specialist

    _____ c) junior stylist

    _____ d) salon manager

7. It is best to get a position in a salon that is above your level of experience so you can receive a bigger paycheck.

    _____ True

    _____ False

8. Cosmetology is a _____ business that revolves around serving clients.

9. List the most important things to remember when servicing your clients:

    a) _____   e) _____

    b) _____   f) _____

    c) _____   g) _____

    d) _____

10. List the habits of successful team players:

    a) _____   e) _____

    b) _____   f) _____

    c) _____   g) _____

    d) _____   h) _____

11. A _____ is a document that outlines all the duties and responsibilities of a particular

    position in a salon or spa.

12. If the salon does not use job descriptions, you may want to _____

    _____ .

13. The three standard methods of compensation for salon professionals are:

    _____ .

14. In addition to a regular salary, it is customary for salon professionals to receive _____ .

    from satisfied clients.

15. To be compensated with a _____ is usually the best way for a new salon professional to start

    out since he or she will most likely not have an established clientele to service.

16. Salaries can be paid in two ways, either on a _____ or an _____ .

17. Being paid a flat rate means _____

    _____ .

18. Being paid by the hour means _____

    _____ .

19. A _____ is a percentage of the money that the salon takes in from

    its sales and is usually offered to stylists once they have built up a loyal clientele.

20. In a _____ structure you receive both a salary and a commission.

    This is commonly used during the transition from junior stylist to full-time stylist or to motivate stylists

    to perform more services.

21. An _____ is the best way to keep tabs on your progress and to get

    feedback from your salon manager and from key and trusted coworkers.

22. On of the best ways to improve your performance is to find someone who is having the kind of success

    you wish to have and use that person as a _____ .

23. When seeking out a role model, observe the stylists who are really good and determine:

a) _____

b) _____

c) _____

d) _____

e) _____

f) _____

g) _____

h) _____

MANAGING YOUR MONEY

24. It is important for professional cosmetologists to create and follow financial plans to ensure the following:

a) _____

b) _____

c) _____

25. In addition to making money, responsible adults are also concerned with _____

_____.

26. Debt can be in the form of _____.

27. What is a personal budget?

_____

28. How can you generate greater income for yourself?

a) _____

b) _____

c) _____

d) _____

29. To get help with your personal finances you should seek the advice of a professional _____

_____ , who will be able to give you advice on reducing your credit card debt, investing

your money, and retirement options.

DISCOVER THE SELLING YOU

30. The practice of recommending and selling additional services to your clients is called_____

_____ .

31. _____ is the act of recommending and selling products to your clients for

at-home hair, skin, and nail care.

32. To be successful in sales, you need _____ .

33. List the 8 principles of selling:

a) _____

_____

b) _____

_____

c) _____

_____

d) _____

_____

e) _____

_____

f) _____

_____

g) _____

_____

h) _____

_____

34. What are the three most common reasons people purchase and consume beauty products?

    _____

35. How can you get the conversation started on retailing products?

    a) _____

    b) _____

    c) _____

    d) _____

    e) _____

    f) _____

36. A _____ consists of the clients you serve on a regular basis, who

    return to you again and again for your services.

37. What things can you do to build your client base?

    a) _____

    b) _____

    c) _____

    d) _____

    e) _____

38. List at least three marketing techniques that will keep your clients coming back to you for services.

    a) _____

    b) _____

    c) _____

    d) _____

39. The best time to think about getting your client back into the salon is after he or she has just left the
    salon and is happy with the service.

    _____ True

    _____ False

40. List three reasons to rebook clients before they leave the salon.

a) _____

b) _____

c) _____

FINAL REVIEW EXAMINATIONS

MULTIPLE CHOICE OR SELECTION

TEST 1: MULTIPLE CHOICE OR SELECTION TEST

DIRECTIONS: Carefully read each statement. Write the letter representing the word or phrase that correctly completes the statement on the blank line to the right of the statement.

1. Using cosmetics to create a new image for a client is one of the services of a:

   a) hairstylist   b) massage therapist
   c) manicurist   d) makeup artist   _____

2. Aromatherapy, hydrotherapy, and massage treatments are often offered by:

   a) nail salons   b) diet centers
   c) day spas   d) barbershops   _____

3. Paying salon bills and taxes is usually *not* one of the duties assigned to the:

   a) accountant   b) salon manager
   c) salon owner   d) entry-level cosmetologist   _____

4. You need commitment to achieve:

   a) perfection   b) popularity
   c) true professionalism   d) mediocrity   _____

5. Taking deep breaths is a useful technique to:

   a) hyperventilate   b) raise your blood pressure
   c) stay calm under stress   d) talk more, listen less   _____

6. Taking care of yourself in a profession like cosmetology:

   a) shows disrespect   b) takes too much time
   c) is self-centered   d) prevents stress and burnout _____

7. Yoga is *not* an activity that involves:

   a) flexibility enhancement   b) stretching exercises
   c) mind and body   d) aerobic exercises   _____

8. Clean, fresh-smelling, and well-maintained clothes are part of:

   a) ergonomics   b) good personal grooming
   c) good posture   d) a healthy mind   _____

9. Accentuating your best features and masking the worst is important when:

   a) selecting shoes   b) reducing stress
   c) applying makeup   d) choosing a client's hairstyle _____

10. Allowing extra time for a consultation is particularly important:

   a)   for a repeat customer
   b)   for clients with high-maintenance styles
   c)   when scheduling a new client
   d)   for every other appointment   _____

11. A consultation card is used primarily to:

   a)   save new styles you like
   b)   schedule reminder calls
   c)   record information from the consultation
   d)   send birthday wishes   _____

12. Hairstyling books and a portfolio are two of the items that are helpful for:

   a)   understanding the total look concept
   b)   preparing for a client consultation
   c)   selling your client on the latest style
   d)   skin care consultation   _____

13. Pathogenic bacteria are:

   a)   harmless
   b)   unimportant
   c)   helpful
   d)   harmful   _____

14. Certain bacteria form spores with tough outer coverings during their:

   a)   mitosis stage
   b)   vegetative stage
   c)   inactive stage
   d)   active stage   _____

15. Disinfected implements should be stored in a container that has:

   a)   been sterilized
   b)   been washed
   c)   been disinfected
   d)   never been used   _____

16. An effective disinfectant solution is required when using:

   a)   bead sterilizers
   b)   autoclaves
   c)   UV sanitizers
   d)   ultrasonic bath cleaners   _____

17. Disinfectants are too strong to use on:

   a)   shampoo bowls
   b)   haircutting tools
   c)   manicure implements
   d)   skin, hair, or nails   _____

18. A Material Safety Data Sheet on every product used in the cosmetology school or salon is required by:

   a)   federal law
   b)   state law
   c)   most instructors
   d)   school regulations   _____

19. The only device among the following that can be used to disinfect implements is the:

   a)   bead sterilizer
   b)   draining basket
   c)   UV sanitizer
   d)   wet sanitizer   _____

20. Infrared lamps should be operated for an exposure time of about:

   a)   30 minutes
   b)   10 minutes
   c)   12 minutes
   d)   5 minutes   _____

21. Of the two electrodes used in electrotherapy, the anode is:

   a) the negative electrode   b) marked with a minus (-) sign
   c) usually black   d) the positive electrode   _____

22. An atom is the smallest particle of a/an _____ that still retains the properties of that _____.

   a) element   b) compound molecule
   c) chemical compounds   d) physical mixture   _____

23. 35% of natural sunlight is made up of:

   a) ultraviolet rays   b) infrared rays
   c) invisible rays   d) visible light   _____

24. The Tesla high-frequency current:

   a) causes chemical changes   b) produces muscle contractions
   c) is a thermal current   d) uses two electrodes   _____

25. With a galvanic current, contraction of the blood vessels is one of the effects of the:

   a) violet ray   b) anode
   c) cathode   d) negative pole   _____

26. A change in the physical properties of a substance without the formation of a new substance is:

   a) a chemical reaction   b) the result of a chemical reaction
   c) a chemical change   d) a physical change   _____

27. Hydrogen ions and hydroxide ions are the products of the ionization of:

   a) oil   b) alcohol
   c) pure water   d) nonaqueous solutions   _____

28. The four most important factors in a hair analysis are texture, density, porosity, and:

   a) hairline   b) length
   c) color   d) elasticity   _____

29. Porosity is defined as the hair's:

   a) ability to stretch   b) ability to absorb moisture
   c) thickness or thinness   d) degree of straightness or curliness   _____

30. The average daily rate of hair loss is:

   a) 5 to 10 hairs   b) 20 to 25 hairs
   c) 35 to 40 hairs   d) 150 to 200 hairs   _____

31. The cortex is the part of the hair in which changes take place during oxidation haircoloring, permanent waving, and:

   a) combing   b) wet setting
   c) brushing   d) cutting   _____

32. The follicle is the tube-like depression in the skin that contains the:

   a)   hair shaft
   b)   sebaceous gland
   c)   cuticle
   d)   hair root
   _____

33. Pityriasis capitis simplex is marked by:

   a)   painful lesions
   b)   dry dandruff
   c)   itch mites
   d)   waxy dandruff
   _____

34. Scabies is a contagious skin disease caused by:

   a)   the itch mite
   b)   bacteria
   c)   head lice
   d)   a fungus
   _____

35. An infestation of the hair and scalp with head lice is called:

   a)   pityriasis capitis simplex
   b)   tinea capitis
   c)   scabies
   d)   pediculosis capitis
   _____

36. The client's skin tone is a consideration when choosing:

   a)   new haircolor
   b)   shape of style
   c)   wave pattern
   d)   point of emphasis
   _____

37. Chemicals can be used to alter:

   a)   facial shape
   b)   wave patterns
   c)   skin tone
   d)   hair texture
   _____

38. In order to balance facial features, you might:

   a)   use cookie cutter design
   b)   suggest makeup instead of hairstyling
   c)   try emphasizing unattractive features
   d)   use asymmetrical hair design
   _____

39. The three basic profiles are concave, convex, and:

   a)   asymmetrical
   b)   straight
   c)   prominent
   d)   concise
   _____

40. The three zones of the face for design purposes are forehead to eyebrows, eyebrows to end of nose, and:

   a)   ear to ear
   b)   forehead to end of nose
   c)   end of nose to bottom of chin
   d)   nose to upper lip
   _____

41. A scalp conditioner is useful for a client with:

   a)   dry hair
   b)   hair loss
   c)   a dry scalp
   d)   an infectious disease
   _____

42. To penetrate the hair cortex, use:

   a)   vigorous brushing
   b)   surfactants
   c)   quaternary ammonium compounds
   d)   concentrated protein conditioner
   _____

43. Humectants are ingredients in conditioners that:

    a) bulk up the hair   b) promote the retention of moisture
    c) reduce frizz   d) penetrate the cortex
                                                                            _____

44. For elderly clients who are experiencing discomfort at the shampoo bowl, recommend:

    a) medicated shampoo   b) staying home
    c) neck padding   d) a dry shampoo
                                                                            _____

45. Acidity and alkalinity are measured by:

    a) pH levels   b) acid precipitation
    c) thermometers   d) barometers
                                                                            _____

46. The angle at which the hair is wrapped determines the:

    a) base size   b) base direction
    c) base control   d) base section
                                                                            _____

47. Base sections are usually the length and width of the:

    a) end paper   b) panel
    c) comb   d) perm tool
                                                                            _____

48. The size of the curl is determined by the:

    a) method of wrapping   b) amount of perm solution
    c) base direction   d) size of the perm tool
                                                                            _____

49. Through a chemical reaction called reduction, permanent waving solution breaks the:

    a) sulfur bonds   b) hydrogen bonds
    c) disulfide bonds   d) salt bonds
                                                                            _____

50. Concave rods have a:

    a) smaller circumference in the center b) greater length than other rods
    c) stiff wire inside   d) uniform circumference along
                                                their length
                                                                            _____

51. To control hair ends when winding the hair on perm tools, use:

    a) absorbent cotton   b) more waving solution
    c) bobby pins   d) end papers
                                                                            _____

52. The hair is wrapped at an angle other than perpendicular to the length of the tool in the technique called:

    a) convex wrapping   b) croquignole wrapping
    c) concave wrapping   d) spiral wrapping
                                                                            _____

53. To properly process resistant hair when permanent waving, it is particularly important to:

    a) saturate it thoroughly   b) use a weaker solution
    c) apply the solution quickly   d) apply solution only once
                                                                            _____

54. Resistant hair that resists penetration by chemicals has:

    a)   a strong cortex   b)   a weak cuticle

    c)   no cuticle   d)   a strong cuticle   _____

55. The strongest side bonds are the:

    a)   peptide bonds   b)   hydrogen bonds

    c)   disulfide bonds   d)   salt bonds   _____

56. Complementary colors are a ____ positioned opposite each other on the color wheel.

    a)   primary and secondary color   b)   dark and light color

    c)   secondary and tertiary color   d)   primary and tertiary color   _____

57. Hair with low porosity has:

    a)   no cuticle   b)   a tight cuticle

    c)   a slightly raised cuticle   d)   a lifted cuticle   _____

58. The hair texture likely to take color faster than the others is:

    a)   coarse hair   b)   medium hair

    c)   thick hair   d)   fine hair   _____

59. The haircolor that is also called "deposit-only haircolor" is:

    a)   demipermanent haircolor   b)   temporary haircolor

    c)   metallic haircolor   d)   semipermanent haircolor   _____

60. The measure of the potential oxidation of varying strengths of hydrogen peroxide is:

    a)   level   b)   volume

    c)   intensity   d)   percentage   _____

61. Bleaching or decolorizing is also called:

    a)   uncoloring   b)   lightening

    c)   stripping   d)   lowlighting   _____

62. The lightness or darkness of color is measured in terms of:

    a)   tone   b)   level

    c)   contributing pigment   d)   intensity   _____

63. The term *tone* or *tonality* is used to describe a color's:

    a)   intensity   b)   level

    c)   warmth or coolness   d)   predominant tonality   _____

64. During haircoloring, coarse hair:

    a)   has tightly grouped melanin granules   b)   has an average response to color

    c)   takes color more quickly   d)   may take longer to process   _____

65. One of the roles of the alkalizing agent in permanent haircolors and lighteners is to:

    a) seal the hair cuticle   b) diffuse through the hair
    c) break up the melanin   d) raise the hair cuticle   _____

66. Basal cell carcinoma is a type of:

    a) skin cancer   b) pigmentation disorder
    c) viral infection   d) bacterial infection   _____

67. Oily, shiny skin indicates the presence of:

    a) psoriasis   b) miliaria rubra
    c) seborrhea   d) asteatosis   _____

68. Blood vessels and capillaries become overdilated because of:

    a) high alcohol intake   b) poor diet
    c) lack of exercise   d) smoking   _____

69. Whiteheads are also called:

    a) comedones   b) milia
    c) miliaria rubra   d) seborrhea   _____

70. The disorder characterized by foul-smelling perspiration is called:

    a) miliaria rubra   b) bromhidrosis
    c) hyperhidrosis   d) anhidrosis   _____

71. A cyst is a type of:

    a) hypertrophy   b) sweat gland disorder
    c) primary lesion   d) secondary lesion   _____

72. The technical term for freckles is:

    a) keratomas   b) lentigines
    c) melanomas   d) verrucas   _____

73. Substances in enzyme peels that help speed up the breakdown of keratin, the protein in skin, are:

    a) salicylic acid   b) keratolytic enzymes
    c) aluminum chloride   d) alphahydroxy acids   _____

74. Fresheners, or skin freshening lotions:

    a) are used on normal skin   b) have a high alcohol content
    c) are used on acne-prone skin   d) have the lowest alcohol content   _____

75. Almond meal or jojoba bead scrubs are products used for:

    a) custom-designed masks   b) gommage
    c) mechanical exfoliation   d) chemical exfoliation   _____

76. An ingredient in some masks that is effective at reducing the production of sebum is:

   a) treatment cream

   b) paraffin

   c) sulfur

   d) pancreatin

   _____

77. Ready-to-use masks that absorb sebum and temporarily contract the pores of the skin are:

   a) clay masks

   b) modelage masks

   c) paraffin masks

   d) keratolytic masks

   _____

78. Foundation is used to:

   a) add a matte finish to the face

   b) give a natural-looking glow to the face

   c) add color to the skin

   d) even skin tone and color

   _____

79. Eye makeup colors that are orange-based are recommended for:

   a) green eyes

   b) blue eyes

   c) brown eyes

   d) all eye colors

   _____

80. A type of foundation that is moist when applied but dries to a powdery finish is:

   a) powder foundation

   b) cream-to-powder foundation

   c) liquid foundation

   d) cream foundation

   _____

81. Face powder that does not change color when applied is:

   a) translucent

   b) loose

   c) pressed

   d) tinted

   _____

82. Face powder is used to:

   a) give a natural-looking glow to the face

   b) even skin tone and color

   c) creates more attractive facial contours

   d) set the foundation

   _____

83. The nail plate, or nail body, rests on and is attached to the:

   a) nail bed

   b) mantle

   c) nail folds

   d) free edge

   _____

84. A nail disorder, usually not reversible, in which the eponychium grows forward and adheres to the nail surface is called:

   a) pterygium

   b) onychatrophia

   c) onychauxis

   d) tile-shaped nails

   _____

85. An inflammation of the matrix bed of the nail with formation of pus and shedding of the nail is:

   a) paronychia

   b) onychia

   c) onychomadesis

   d) onycholysis

   _____

86. Pyogenic granuloma is a severe nail inflammation characterized by a growth of:

    a)　brown fungus　　　　　　　b)　excess cuticle
    c)　excess nail　　　　　　　　d)　red tissue　　　　　_____

87. A disease caused by vegetable parasites is:

    a)　paronychia　　　　　　　　b)　pterygium
    c)　onychosis　　　　　　　　　d)　tinea　　　　　_____

88. Nail diseases that involve the shedding of the nail include all the following *except*:

    a)　onycholysis　　　　　　　　b)　onychoptosis
    c)　onychomadesis　　　　　　　d)　onychia　　　　　_____

89. Ringworm is technically known as:

    a)　onychocryptosis　　　　　　b)　tinea
    c)　agnail　　　　　　　　　　　d)　onychia　　　　　_____

90. A rate of nail growth of ⅛ inch per month is average for:

    a)　infants　　　　　　　　　　b)　elderly persons
    c)　children　　　　　　　　　　d)　normal adults　　　　　_____

91. Many small businesses fail because their plans are not well matched to their:

    a)　capital　　　　　　　　　　b)　color scheme
    c)　personnel　　　　　　　　　d)　parking space　　　　　_____

92. Documents that must be retained for at least seven years, largely for tax purposes, include all the following *except*:

    a)　payroll books　　　　　　　b)　canceled checks
    c)　yearly records　　　　　　　d)　salon brochures　　　　　_____

93. Good plumbing and lighting are essential for:

    a)　high visibility　　　　　　　b)　effective retailing
    c)　satisfactory client services　　d)　positive manager-employee
    　　　　　　　　　　　　　　　　　　relations　　　　　_____

94. The salon receptionist is in charge of:

    a)　coordinating daily schedules　　b)　servicing clients
    c)　sanitation and disinfection　　　d)　general operations　　　　　_____

95. A salon owned and managed by a hairstylist is considered a:

    a)　franchise salon　　　　　　　b)　small independent salon
    c)　chain salon　　　　　　　　　d)　booth rental establishment　　　　　_____

96. In a true/false test, keep in mind that:

    a)　choose the statement with all or none　　b)　the entire statement must be true
    c)　some of it should be true　　　　　　　d)　select the shorter statement　　　　　_____

97. Observing the operations of local salons is part of:

    a)   developing a resume   b)   spying

    c)   licensing   d)   networking   _____

98. In a profession with irregular income like the beauty industry, to ensure that you always have enough:

    a)   never take time off   b)   save every penny

    c)   stick to a budget   d)   insist on straight salary   _____

99. The first step in selling is to:

    a)   tell clients what they need   b)   be aggressive

    c)   exaggerate product claims   d)   sell yourself   _____

100. The steady customers whom you serve on a regular basis are considered your:

    a)   client base   b)   clientele

    c)   clinicians   d)   basic clients   _____

TEST II: MULTIPLE CHOICE OR SELECTION TEST

DIRECTIONS: Carefully read each statement. Write the letter representing the word or phrase that correctly completes the statement on the blank line to the right of the statement.

1. A wig specialist may find it gratifying to work with:

   a) cancer patients   b) clients who need nail tips
   c) clients desiring new wave patterns   d) clients desiring new haircolor   _____

2. As early as the glacial age, people have been practicing the skills of:

   a) nail enhancements   b) haircutting and hairstyling
   c) permanent waving   d) dentistry   _____

3. The ancient Egyptians were the first people to:

   a) use cosmetics   b) make implements from bone
   c) bury their dead   d) use barber poles   _____

4. Ethics can be defined as:

   a) moral principles   b) building character
   c) perfectionism   d) guidelines for success   _____

5. In order to act professionally, we need to:

   a) get ahead of our coworkers   b) understand the needs of others
   c) always be in the right   d) keep to ourselves   _____

6. The technique of agreeing and asking what you can do to remedy the situation is effective
   with:

   a) an unreasonable supervisor   b) a difficult, disgruntled client
   c) a dishonest coworker   d) an aggressive vendor   _____

7. Personal hygiene involves the daily practice of:

   a) dressing for the occasion   b) applying tasteful makeup
   c) eating healthy food   d) cleanliness and health   _____

8. The Old English word for "whole" is:

   a) *halala*   b) *halos*
   c) *hal*   d) *haiku*   _____

9. The proper functioning of our organs is enhanced by:

   a) a sedentary lifestyle   b) a high intake of salt
   c) regular physical exercise   d) a demanding job   _____

10. Clarification with the client will aid in:

    a) distraction   b) communication
    c) creating a dramatic look   d) establishing a styling regimen   _____

11. The person with a classic style chooses clothing that is:

   a)   ornate and daring   b)   dull and drab
   c)   simple and sophisticated   d)   very trendy   _____

12. Use of a mirror is one of the first steps in a:

   a)   consultation   b)   pedicure
   c)   shampoo   d)   scalp massage   _____

13. In the salon, the constant use of antibacterial soaps:

   a)   is beneficial to the skin   b)   is required by the EPA
   c)   is required for ahnd-washing d)   may lead to skin problems   _____

14. Saprophytes are bacteria that live on:

   a)   an animal host   b)   molds and mildews
   c)   dead matter   d)   living matter   _____

15. Disease in plant or animal tissue is caused by:

   a)   nonpathogenic bacteria   b)   saprophytes
   c)   pathogenic bacteria   d)   acidophilus   _____

16. Mitosis is the process by which bacteria:

   a)   move about   b)   release toxins
   c)   divide   d)   become inactive   _____

17. The HIV virus is *not* transmitted:

   a)   by IV users sharing needles b)   by kissing or hugging
   c)   through cuts and sores   d)   through unprotected sexual contact _____

18. There are three main levels of decontamination:

   a)   disinfection, scrubbing, sanitation   b)   sterilization, disinfection, sanitation
   c)   sterilization, cleaning, sanitation   d)   steam autoclave, dry heat,
                                                     disinfection   _____

19. The type of bacteria that has a rod shape is called:

   a)   spirilla   b)   diplococci
   c)   staphylococci   d)   bacilli   _____

20. It is estimated that 1 in five Americans will develop skin cancer, and _____ of those cancers
    will be the result of exposure to UV radiation from the sun and from tanning beds.

   a)   10%   b)   25%
   c)   90%   d)   50%   _____

21. Oxidation occurs when a substance is combined with:

   a)   nitrogen   b)   hydrogen
   c)   pure water   d)   oxygen   _____

22. Because of the ionization of water, _____ is possible.

    a)　oxidation
    b)　pH
    c)　combustion
    d)　reduction
    _____

23. The branch of science that studies substances containing carbon is:

    a)　inorganic chemistry
    b)　organic chemistry
    c)　myology
    d)　physics
    _____

24. Safety precautions for using electrical equipment include all the following *except*:

    a)　handle equipment with dry hands
    b)　use only one plug per outlet
    c)　inspect equipment regularly
    d)　disconnect equipment by pulling the cord
    _____

25. An example of a chemical compound is:

    a)　pure water (H_2O)
    b)　salt water
    c)　pure air
    d)　concrete
    _____

26. The main characteristic of miscible liquids is that they:

    a)　separate easily over time
    b)　can be mixed together without separating
    c)　require surfactants to mix together
    d)　are not capable of being mixed
    _____

27. Two or more immiscible substances united with the aid of a binder are called a/an:

    a)　suspension
    b)　emulsion
    c)　solution
    d)　chemical compound
    _____

28. Side bonds account for the hair's:

    a)　color
    b)　elasticity
    c)　fragility
    d)　porosity
    _____

29. Fragilitas crinium is characterized by:

    a)　split ends
    b)　dry dandruff
    c)　brittle hair
    d)　ringworm
    _____

30. The bond that joins the sulfur atoms of two neighboring cysteine amino acids to create cystine is the:

    a)　peptide bond
    b)　salt bond
    c)　hydrogen bond
    d)　disulfide bond
    _____

31. A generalized thinning of hair in the crown area is characteristic of:

    a)　androgenic alopecia in men
    b)　alopecia areata in men
    c)　alopecia areata in women
    d)　androgenic alopecia in women
    _____

32. *Trichorrhexis nodosa* is the technical term for:

    a)   beaded hair   b)   brittle hair

    c)   knotted hair   d)   abnormal hair growth   _____

33. Permanent haircolors, perm solutions, and chemical relaxers must have an alkaline pH in order to:

    a)   remove the cuticle layer   b)   remove the cortex

    c)   penetrate the cuticle layer   d)   penetrate the medulla   _____

34. The hair bulb fits over and covers the:

    a)   follicle   b)   hair shaft

    c)   dermal papilla   d)   arrector pili   _____

35. Peptide bonds are the chemical bonds that join:

    a)   polypeptide chains together   b)   salt bonds together

    c)   sulfur atoms together   d)   amino acids to each other   _____

36. The position and prominence of facial bones determines:

    a)   hair type   b)   coloring

    c)   hairline   d)   facial shape   _____

37. There are many more styling choices available today for:

    a)   female clients   b)   movie stars

    c)   wealthy clients   d)   male clients   _____

38. Moving the hair forward in the chin area is effective if your client has a:

    a)   concave profile   b)   small nose

    c)   convex profile   d)   large chin   _____

39. Hair cut above or below the chin line will help to balance a:

    a)   prominent nose   b)   large chin

    c)   small chin   d)   large ears   _____

40. Wavy, coarse hair, if not properly shaped, will appear:

    a)   damaged   b)   sleek and smooth

    c)   small and narrow   d)   very wide   _____

41. Natural bristle brushes have overlapping layers that clean and:

    a)   slow down circulation   b)   loosen scales from the scalp

    c)   add luster to the hair   d)   repair split ends   _____

42. A pH range of 4.5 to 5.5 in shampoo is considered:

    a)   too acidic   b)   very alkaline

    c)   acid-balanced   d)   ineffective   _____

43. A protein conditioner is effective for:

    a)   adding some slight color   b)   stimulating blood circulation to the scalp

    c)   slightly increasing hair diameter   d)   even distribution of oil   _____

44. Shampoos that contain acidic ingredients designed to cut through product buildup are called:

    a)   balancing   b)   powder

    c)   nonstripping   d)   clarifying   _____

45. Cleansing the hair and scalp is the primary purpose of:

    a)   shampooing in the salon   b)   the use of conditioners

    c)   an appointment at the salon   d)   a day at the spa   _____

46. Rebuilding broken disulfide bonds and deactivating any remaining waving solution in the hair are the functions of:

    a)   ammonia   b)   activator

    c)   conditioner   d)   neutralizer   _____

47. If permanently waved hair has been overprocessed, it means that:

    a)   too many disulfide bonds have been broken   b)   the hair is always overly curly

    c)   the hair is curlier at the ends   d)   not enough disulfide bonds are broken   _____

48. In terms of chemical texture services, fine hair:

    a)   does not present any problems   b)   is more resistant to processing

    c)   is difficult to penetrate   d)   is easier to process than coarse or medium   _____

49. For spiral wrapping on extremely long hair, the ideal tool is the:

    a)   concave rod   b)   convex rod

    c)   straight rod   d)   circle tool   _____

50. Straight rods have a:

    a)   uniform circumference along their length   b)   smaller circumference at one end

    c)   smaller circumference in the center   d)   smaller circumference at both ends   _____

51. About 1/3 of the hair's total strength comes from:

    a)   peptide bonds   b)   amino acids

    c)   hydrogen bonds   d)   end bonds   _____

52. Chemical texture services permanently alter the hair's natural:

    a)   texture   b)   density

    c)   wave pattern   d)   color   _____

53. In the croquignole wrapping technique, the hair is wrapped:

    a) in partially overlapping layers   b) from scalp to ends

    c) from ends to scalp   d) at an angle other than perpendicular   _____

54. Base control is the position of the perm tool in relation to:

    a) the hair   b) the end papers

    c) its base section   d) the panel   _____

55. It is possible to change the hair's natural wave pattern by breaking the side bonds in the:

    a) medulla   b) cortex

    c) follicle   d) cuticle   _____

56. Mixing equal amounts of two primary colors yields a:

    a) secondary color   b) neutralized color

    c) tertiary color   d) complementary color   _____

57. Creating the correct degree of contributing pigment is the goal of:

    a) toning   b) permanent coloring

    c) lowlighting   d) decolorizing   _____

58. An example of a natural haircolor is:

    a) metallic haircolor   b) hydrogen peroxide

    c) henna   d) aniline derivatives   _____

59. Haircolors can be divided into four general categories based partly on how long they last, which is affected by:

    a) the client's hair type   b) their retail price

    c) their chemical composition   d) the developer strength   _____

60. Eumelanin gives the hair:

    a) white color   b) blonde color

    c) black and brown color   d) red color   _____

61. A developer supplies _____ to develop color molecules and create a change in hair color.

    a) hydrogen   b) nitrogen

    c) sulfur   d) oxygen   _____

62. The primary colors are red, yellow, and:

    a) black   b) green

    c) orange   d) blue   _____

63. The predominant tonality of an existing color is called its:

    a) contributing pigment   b) intensity

    c) base color   d) level   _____

64. The type of haircolor that has only a coating action on the hair is:

    a) temporary haircolor   b) demipermanent haircolor
    c) semipermanent haircolor   d) permanent haircolor   _____

65. Contributing pigment is exposed when you:

    a) glaze the hair   b) use demipermanent color
    c) process with permanent haircolor d) lighten natural hair color   _____

66. The nervous system controls the excretion of sweat from the body, at the daily rate of:

    a) 1 to 2 quarts   b) 1 to 2 pints
    c) 1 to 2 cups   d) 1 to 2 tablespoons   _____

67. The fatty or oily substance that lubricates the skin is secreted by:

    a) hair follicles   b) sebaceous glands
    c) sudoriferous glands   d) sweat pores   _____

68. The fatty layer below the dermis is called:

    a) collagen layer   b) reticular layer
    c) papillary layer   d) subcutaneous tissue   _____

69. A tumor is an abnormal:

    a) cell mass   b) skin pigmentation
    c) accumulation of fluid   d) secondary lesion   _____

70. Chloasma is also known as moth patches or:

    a) freckles   b) calluses
    c) liver spots   d) birthmarks   _____

71. One of the functions of blood and lymph is to:

    a) supply nourishment to the skin   b) protect skin cells from UV rays
    c) lubricate the skin   d) make the skin waterproof   _____

72. Contraction and weakening of blood vessels and small capillaries is caused by:

    a) alcohol   b) excess protein
    c) nicotine   d) lack of exercise   _____

73. A type of enzyme peel that stays soft during application rather than drying to a crust uses:

    a) a powdered enzyme   b) oatmeal granules
    c) a cream solution   d) plant-derived acids   _____

74. Gommage is a combination of mechanical peeling and:

    a) alphahydroxy acids   b) crystals
    c) gums   d) an enzyme   _____

75. Ampules are sealed glass vials containing single applications of:

    a) moisturizer   b) treatment cream
    c) concentrated extracts   d) exfoliant   _____

76. If a client does not first use an alphahydroxy product at home for two weeks, an alpha
    hydroxy exfoliation in the salon may:

    a) cause an allergic reaction   b) cause discomfort
    c) have no effect   d) exfoliate too deeply   _____

77. To keep paraffin and gypsum/plaster masks from sticking to the skin, you may use:

    a) gauze   b) powder
    c) plastic wrap   d) oil   _____

78. Matching the color of the eye shadow to the color of the eyes:

    a) enhances eye color   b) creates a flat field of color
    c) creates a desirable daytime look   d) creates a dramatic look   _____

79. A cosmetic that helps keep lip color from feathering is:

    a) powder   b) foundation
    c) lip liner   d) concealer   _____

80. To fill in sparse areas of the eyebrows, use:

    a) mascara   b) eye shadow
    c) eyebrow color   d) liquid eyeliner   _____

81. The cosmetic used to outline and emphasize the eyes is:

    a) mascara   b) eyebrow pencil
    c) eyeliner   d) highlight color   _____

82. Cheek color is also called blush, blusher, or:

    a) cheek shadow   b) pancake makeup
    c) rouge   d) tinted moisturizer   _____

83. A bacteria that can cause nail infections when artificial products such as tips and wraps
    are applied under unsanitary conditions is:

    a) Treponema pallida   b) Mycobacterium fortuitum furunculosis
    c) Pseudomonas aeruginosa   d) Borrelia burgdorferi   _____

84. Paronychia, which affects the tissues surrounding the nail, is a/an:

    a) periodic shedding of the nail   b) ingrown nail
    c) loosening of the nail   d) bacterial inflammation   _____

85. Leukonychia is characterized by:

    a) wasting away of the nail   b) overgrowth of the nail
    c) white spots on the nail   d) split cuticles

86. Onychocryptosis is commonly called:

    a)   bitten nails   b)   felon
    c)   ringworm   d)   ingrown nails   _____

87. Whitish patches that can be scraped off the nail surface are characteristic of a common
    form of:

    a)   pyogenic granuloma   b)   tinea unguium
    c)   felon   d)   onychoptosis   _____

88. The matrix bed (nail root) is composed of matrix cells that produce the:

    a)   hyponychium   b)   eponychium
    c)   mantle   d)   nail plate   _____

89. Poor blood circulation or a heart disorder can sometimes cause:

    a)   hangnails   b)   leukonychia
    c)   onychophagy   d)   blue nails   _____

90. The bacteria called *Pseudomonas aeruginosa*:

    a)   is difficult to kill   b)   cannot live in the presence of oxygen
    c)   thrives in aerobic conditions   d)   is very rare   _____

91. Your local (city) officials are the people you must contact about:

    a)   Social Security   b)   sales taxes
    c)   building renovations   d)   licenses   _____

92. A perpetual inventory helps to prevent:

    a)   overstocking or shortage of supplies   b)   overcharging by suppliers
    c)   reliance on client cards   d)   theft of supplies   _____

93. A central location in the salon is the best place to keep:

    a)   consumption supplies   b)   client records
    c)   business records   d)   cash receipts   _____

94. Demographics that would be helpful in choosing a location for a salon include information
    about a specific population's size, average income, and:

    a)   political affiliations   b)   dietary habits
    c)   buying habits   d)   religious preferences   _____

95. As you move into the workplace, you'll be rewarded for:

    a)   arrogance   b)   hard work
    c)   tardiness   d)   self-interest   _____

96. Skimming the entire test before you begin:

    a)   wastes time   b)   is cheating
    c)   slows you down   d)   is a helpful test-taking strategy   _____

97. Developing a detailed vocabulary list, reviewing past quizzes, and keeping a well-organized notebook are all part of:

    a)   test preparation   b)   deductive reasoning

    c)   creating a portfolio   d)   writing a resume   _____

98. Knowing your products is a principle of:

    a)   budgeting   b)   salon teamwork

    c)   financial planning   d)   successful sales   _____

99. Asking your clients what they use to shampoo, condition, and style their hair is:

    a)   an upselling technique   b)   a waste of time

    c)   disrespectful   d)   a retailing technique   _____

100. Reportable income for tax purposes includes all the following *except*:

    a)   school loans   b)   salary

    c)   commission   d)   tips   _____

TEST III: MULTIPLE CHOICE OR SELECTION TEST

DIRECTIONS: Carefully read each statement. Write the letter representing the word or phrase that correctly completes the statement on the blank line to the right of the statement.

1. The job of entry-level salon stylist is usually offered to a:

   a)   cosmetic chemist   b)   new cosmetology graduate

   c)   salon manager   d)   haircolor specialist   _____

2. Standards for the cosmetology industry are set by:

   a)   professional associations   b)   salon owners

   c)   cosmetic companies   d)   government regulatory agencies   _____

3. There is evidence that nail care was practiced in Egypt and China as early as:

   a)   1400 A.D.   b)   3000 B.C.

   c)   500 B.C.   d)   500 A.D.   _____

4. Expressing our emotions in an appropriate manner is related to our level of:

   a)   motivation   b)   emotional stability

   c)   career skills   d)   productivity   _____

5. The state licensing boards set the:

   a)   location of new salons   b)   fee structures

   c)   guidelines for new styles   d)   code of ethics   _____

6. Looking ahead toward your goals helps keep you:

   a)   dissatisfied   b)   overwhelmed

   c)   motivated   d)   discouraged   _____

7. To prevent a variety of illnesses, you should:

   a)   read medical books   b)   eat fast foods

   c)   eat a healthy, nutritious diet   d)   follow the latest fad diet   _____

8. Measures that help prevent physical strain include all of the following *except*:

   a)   swiveling the client's chair   b)   twisting your body when reaching

   c)   keeping your shears sharpened   d)   keeping your back straight   _____

9. Your outward appearance and conduct are part of your:

   a)   code of ethics   b)   professional image

   c)   personal hygiene   d)   technical skills   _____

10. One task you can always perform that will help you build good client relationships is:

   a)   making decisions for your clients   b)   keeping accurate consultation cards

   c)   never falling behind   d)   playing therapist for your clients   _____

11. The main purpose of the consultation is to:

    a) gather information   b) focus on any damage
    c) lecture the client   d) sell your services   _____

12. The amount of time a client has for style maintenance is related to:

    a) lifestyle   b) hair type
    c) wave pattern   d) income   _____

13. The bacteria with a corkscrew or spiral shape are:

    a) bacilli   b) spirilla
    c) staphylococci   d) diplococci   _____

14. *Mycobacterium fortuitum furunculosis* is a:

    a) rod-shaped bacteria   b) spiral-shaped bacteria
    c) corkscrew-shaped bacteria   d) round bacteria   _____

15. Syphilis is an example of a/an:

    a) subjective symptom   b) general infection
    c) epidemic   d) local infection   _____

16. Penetrating cells and becoming part of them is characteristic of:

    a) bacteria   b) parasites
    c) fungi   d) viruses   _____

17. Contaminants in a salon include:

    a) phenols and quats   b) EPA-registered disinfectants
    c) makeup on a clean towel   d) bactericides and fungicides _____

18. Pus-forming bacteria called streptococci cause:

    a) Lyme disease   b) pneumonia
    c) boils   d) strep throat   _____

19. Parasites are a type of:

    a) disease   b) pathogenic virus
    c) pathogenic bacteria   d) nonpathogenic bacteria   _____

20. An example of matter changing from a liquid form to a gas is:

    a) water freezing   b) steam condensing
    c) water boiling   d) ice melting   _____

21. Alkanolamines are often used in hair products in place of:

    a) peroxide   b) ammonia
    c) aniline dye   d) alcohol   _____

22. Plastics, gasoline, and pesticides are all examples of:

   a) inorganic substances   b) substances lacking carbon
   c) organic substances   d) nonflammable substances   _____

23. The unit that measures the strength of an electric current (the number of electrons flowing through a wire) is the:

   a) watt   b) volt
   c) ampere   d) ohm   _____

24. The electrotherapy treatment called desincrustation:

   a) is done with a high-frequency current   b) is used to treat acne and comedones
   c) causes muscular contractions   d) is done with a faradic current   _____

25. In the event of electrical overload, a circuit breaker:

   a) switch from DC to AC   b) produce different types of electric currents

   c) interrupts or shuts off an electric circuit   d) melts or blows out   _____

26. A direct current (DC):

   a) is rapid and interrupted   b) is used in faradic treatments
   c) produces a chemical reaction d) produces a mechanical reaction   _____

27. The least penetrating invisible rays are:

   a) infrared rays   b) white rays
   c) combination light rays   d) ultraviolet rays   _____

28. The two main divisions of the hair are the hair shaft and the:

   a) follicle   b) arrector pili
   c) bulb   d) hair root   _____

29. Clients should be referred to a physician if they show signs of:

   a) pityriasis capitis simplex   b) tinea capitis
   c) trichoptilosis   d) trichorrhexis nodosa   _____

30. Practicing approved sanitation and disinfection procedures is necessary to prevent the spread of:

   a) trichorrhexis nodosa   b) androgenic alopecia
   c) tinea and pityriasis   d) monilethrix   _____

31. Postpartum alopecia affects:

   a) women over age 40   b) both men and women
   c) women at the end of a pregnancy   d) men with autoimmune disease   _____

32. An oval cross-section is typical of:

    a)   all hair types   b)   wavy hair

    c)   straight hair   d)   extremely curly hair   _____

33. Previous overprocessing during chemical services can leave the hair:

    a)   resistant   b)   less porous

    c)   overly porous   d)   healthier   _____

34. The three layers of the hair shaft are the cuticle, medulla, and:

    a)   cortex   b)   follicle

    c)   root   d)   bulb   _____

35. A hair stream is:

    a)   hair flowing in opposite directions   b)   hair that forms a circular pattern

    c)   hair flowing in the same direction   d)   a tuft of hair standing straight up   _____

36. The side view of a face or figure is called a:

    a)   front view   b)   profile

    c)   silhouette   d)   bird's-eye view   _____

37. Hair worn full and falling below the jaw works well for a client with a:

    a)   long, narrow nose   b)   square jaw

    c)   wide-set eyes   d)   long jaw   _____

38. Oval is generally considered to be the ideal:

    a)   hair color   b)   nose shape

    c)   hairline   d)   facial type   _____

39. A small and narrow silhouette is created by hair that is:

    a)   fine and very curly   b)   coarse and straight

    c)   medium and wavy   d)   fine and straight   _____

40. When styling the hair around the ears, it is important to consider:

    a)   the shape of the eyes   b)   if the client wears glasses

    c)   the shape of the forehead.   d)   the chin line   _____

41. To restore moisture and elasticity to the hair while adding volume, use:

    a)   dry shampoos   b)   clarifying shampoos

    c)   conditioning shampoos   d)   medicated shampoos   _____

42. The condition of the client's hair is a consideration in the:

    a)   inclusion of a scalp massage   b)   selection of shampoo

    c)   method of draping   d)   use of hard or soft water   _____

43. For a client with coarse, wavy hair, all the following products are recommended *except*:

   a)   moisturizing shampoo   b)   leave-in conditioner
   c)   volumizing shampoo   d)   protein treatments   _____

44. When giving a chemical service:

   a)   do not brush the hair   b)   use firm pressure when shampooing
   c)   brush the hair thoroughly   d)   use concentrated protein treatment   _____

45. When deep, penetrating conditioners are applied, it is sometimes necessary to:

   a)   wrap the hair in heated towels   b)   put the client under a hooded dryer
   c)   use a blow-dryer on the hair   d)   rinse and reapply   _____

46. The most important factors to consider in a hair analysis for chemical texture services include:

   a)   elasticity and color   b)   density and length
   c)   length and growth direction   d)   texture and porosity   _____

47. In the first part of any perm, the physical change that occurs when the hair is wrapped on perm rods breaks the:

   a)   peptide bonds   b)   hydrogen bonds
   c)   disulfide bonds   d)   salt bonds   _____

48. Wrapping the hair on base:

   a)   may damage the hair   b)   creates the least volume
   c)   creates minimal volume at the scalp   d)   minimizes stress on the hair   _____

49. Base direction refers to the angle:

   a)   at which the hair is wrapped   b)   of the hair to the length of the tool
   c)   at which the tool is positioned on the head   d)   in which the hair is combed   _____

50. The most common neutralizer for permanent waving is:

   a)   glyceryl monothioglycolate   b)   hydrogen peroxide
   c)   ammonium thioglycolate   d)   ammonia   _____

51. The reducing agents used in permanent waving solutions are:

   a)   hydrogen peroxide   b)   neutralizers
   c)   ammonias   d)   thiol compounds   _____

52. Changes in pH are sufficient to break:

   a)   salt bonds   b)   disulfide bonds
   c)   hydrogen bonds   d)   peptide bonds   _____

53. In the second part of any perm, a chemical change occurs when the permanent waving solution is applied, breaking the:

   a)   disulfide bonds   b)   salt bonds
   c)   polypeptide chains   d)   hydrogen bonds   _____

54. A highly alkaline, or high pH, perm solution is recommended for hair that is:

   a) damaged
   b) chemically treated
   c) resistant
   d) porous   _____

55. *Cold waves* is another term for:

   a) ammonia-free waves
   b) alkaline waves
   c) low-pH waves
   d) acid-balanced waves   _____

56. 40 volume hydrogen peroxide is used to provide:

   a) additional lift with permanent color
   b) standard volume
   c) less lightening to enhance natural color
   d) maximum lift with high-lift colors   _____

57. Permanent haircolor is considered the best product for:

   a) covering gray hair
   b) refreshing faded color
   c) creating fun, temporary results
   d) introducing clients to haircolor   _____

58. The color green is made up of equal amounts of:

   a) orange and violet
   b) yellow and blue
   c) blue and red
   d) red and yellow   _____

59. The haircolor formulated to last only 6 to 8 shampoos is:

   a) temporary haircolor
   b) semipermanent haircolor
   c) demipermanent haircolor
   d) permanent haircolor   _____

60. Hair that takes color quickly and also tends to fade quickly generally has:

   a) high porosity
   b) average porosity
   c) low porosity
   d) no porosity   _____

61. Mixing equal amounts of a secondary color and its neighboring primary color on the color wheel results in a:

   a) warm color
   b) complementary color
   c) tertiary color
   d) secondary color   _____

62. Tertiary colors include:

   a) violet
   b) black
   c) blue-green
   d) orange   _____

63. In haircoloring, hydrogen peroxide is the most commonly used:

   a) dye precursor
   b) oxidizer
   c) alkalizing agent
   d) reducing agent   _____

64. Blue is the:

   a) darkest warm color
   b) medium secondary color
   c) darkest primary color
   d) medium primary color   _____

65. Metallic haircolors change hair color gradually by:

a)   progressive buildup
b)   changing the hair structure
c)   destroying melanin
d)   staining the cortex

_____

66. In its topical form, vitamin A has been shown to:

a)   support the bones of the body
b)   treat different types of acne
c)   heal burns and stretch marks
d)   promote collagen production

_____

67. The nerve fibers in the skin that react to heat, cold, touch, pressure, and pain are the:

a)   autonomic nerves
b)   sensory nerve fibers
c)   motor nerve fibers
d)   secretory nerve fibers

_____

68. Psoriasis is a/an:

a)   non-contagious disease
b)   occupational disorder
c)   disorder of the sebaceous glands
d)   hypertrophy

_____

69. Leukoderma is a skin disorder that is further classified as:

a)   chloasma and stains
b)   vitiligo and albinism
c)   vitiligo and chloasma
d)   nevi and stains

_____

70. The eyelids have the _____ on the body.

a)   thinnest skin
b)   thickest skin
c)   deepest follicles
d)   largest follicles

_____

71. The scalp has the:

a)   thinnest skin
b)   thickest skin
c)   deepest follicles
d)   smallest oil glands

_____

72. A cicatrix is a slightly raised mark on the skin formed after:

a)   the healing of an injury
b)   an insect bite
c)   contact with poison ivy
d)   scratching or scraping

_____

73. A type of facial mask that both warms up and cools down on the skin is the:

a)   paraffin mask
b)   modelage mask
c)   clay mask
d)   custom-designed mask

_____

74. The peeling and shredding of the horny (outer) layer of the skin is called:

a)   freshening
b)   fulling
c)   exfoliation
d)   friction

_____

75. Face wash is best used on clients with:

a)   oily or combination skin
b)   mature skin
c)   dry skin
d)   wrinkled skin

_____

76. Cleansing cream is best used on:

    a) normal skin
    b) oily skin
    c) acne skin
    d) very dry or mature skin   _____

77. A facial product that restores the skin's natural pH after cleansing is:

    a) emollient
    b) treatment cream
    c) tonic lotion
    d) gommage   _____

78. Pressed powder eye shadow may be used with an eyeliner brush to:

    a) color the eyelashes
    b) color the eyebrows
    c) create a softer lined effect
    d) line the lips   _____

79. Lip color should be applied:

    a) with a lip brush
    b) directly from the container
    c) with your little finger
    d) with a spatula   _____

80. Cool colors include:

    a) yellow-greens
    b) red-oranges
    c) most reds
    d) blue-reds   _____

81. The three main factors to consider when choosing makeup colors for a client are skin color, hair color, and:

    a) clothing color
    b) eyebrow color
    c) nail color
    d) eye color   _____

82. Eye shadow that is a contour color is used to:

    a) make an area appear larger
    b) even skin tone on the eye
    c) highlight a specific area
    d) minimize a specific area   _____

83. If a client comes to you with onychophagy:

    a) file the nails down
    b) do not touch the nails
    c) suggest frequent manicures
    d) refer him to a physician   _____

84. The nail bed is the portion of skin:

    a) that surrounds the nail plate
    b) that is most visible
    c) that produces the nail plate
    d) on which the nail plate rests   _____

85. *Onyx* is the technical term for:

    a) nail disease or deformity
    b) the finger
    c) the nail
    d) nail matrix inflammation   _____

86. Tile-shaped nails have an increased crosswise curvature throughout the nail plate caused by an increased curvature in the:

    a) nail grooves
    b) cuticles
    c) matrix bed
    d) free edge   _____

87. The lunula, or half moon, is the visible portion of the:

    a) nail bed   b) matrix bed (nail root)
    c) bed epithelium   d) mantle   _____

88. Specialized ligaments attach the nail bed and matrix bed to the:

    a) underlying bone   b) bed epithelium
    c) blood vessels   d) muscles   _____

89. Careless filing and excessive use of cuticle solvents and nail polish removers are among the causes of:

    a) white spots   b) eggshell nails
    c) bruised nails   d) abnormal nail brittleness   _____

90. Uneven growth of the nails, usually the result of illness or injury, can cause:

    a) corrugations   b) melanonychia
    c) blue nails   d) hangnails   _____

91. When a stylist rents a station in a salon from a salon owner or landlord, it is called:

    a) booth (or chair) rental   b) a partnership
    c) individual ownership   d) upselling   _____

92. At any given time, the appointment book should reflect:

    a) yearly income   b) what is taking place in the salon
    c) retail sales   d) the salon's financial plan   _____

93. In a corporation, ownership is shared by three or more people called:

    a) stockholders   b) partners
    c) sole proprietors   d) joint owners   _____

94. When booking appointments by telephone, if a stylist is not available for the time a client requests, you should first suggest:

    a) calling the client in case of cancellation   b) other times the stylist is available
    c) that the client call back in a few days   d) trying another stylist   _____

95. When writing a resume, do all of the following *except*:

    a) mention hobbies and memberships b) focus on career goals
    c) use action verbs   d) keep it short   _____

96. If asked an improper or illegal question during a job interview, a good response is:

    a) to ignore the question   b) that the question is irrelevant
    c) refuse to answer   d) to threaten a lawsuit   _____

97. During your job search, send a resume and cover letter when you're ready to:

    a) network   b) request an interview
    c) observe a salon   d) take the licensing exam   _____

98. A job description should contain:

    a)   age limitations   b)   all your duties and responsibilities
    c)   problem-solving ideas   d)   a personal budget   _____

99. A method of estimating income and expenses is:

    a)   a mortgage   b)   estimated taxes
    c)   a 401K   d)   a budget   _____

100. When job hunting, finding a salon that matches your personal style is:

    a)   an important factor   b)   too limiting
    c)   unrealistic   d)   disrespectful to employers _____

ANATOMY TEST: MULTIPLE CHOICE OR SELECTION TEST

DIRECTIONS: Carefully read each statement. Write the letter representing the word or phrase that correctly completes the statement on the blank line to the right of the statement.

1. The cervical nerves and their branches affect the muscles of the:

    a)   back of the head and neck   b)   temple and eyebrow

    c)   chin and lower lip   d)   mouth   _____

2. The endocrine system is made up of a group of specialized:

    a)   nerves   b)   joints

    c)   lymph nodes   d)   glands   _____

3. The pericardium is the membrane that encloses the:

    a)   aorta   b)   heart

    c)   ventricles   d)   arteries   _____

4. Cytoplasm is responsible for:

    a)   allowing entry of soluble substances   b)   enclosing the cell

    c)   manufacturing toxins   d)   cell growth and self-repair   _____

5. The central nervous system is composed of the brain and:

    a)   heart   b)   spinal cord

    c)   peripheral nervous system   d)   voluntary muscles   _____

6. The phalanges are the bones of the:

    a)   shoulder   b)   forearm

    c)   wrist   d)   fingers   _____

7. Exocrine glands produce a substance that travels through tube-like:

    a)   enzymes   b)   blood vessels

    c)   ducts   d)   cells   _____

8. The auriculotemporal nerve is a branch of the fifth cranial nerve and affects the:

    a)   point and lower side of the nose   b)   skin of the chin

    c)   external ear and skin above the temple   d)   skin of the lower eyelid   _____

9. The infraorbital artery supplies blood to the:

    a)   muscles of the eye   b)   lower lip

    c)   side and crown of the head   d)   upper eyelid and forehead   _____

10. The adductors are muscles of the hand that:

    a)   straighten the wrist and hand   b)   separate the fingers

    c)   draw the fingers together   d)   bring the thumb toward the fingers _____

11. The orbicularis oculi is a muscle that rings the:

     a)   ear   b)   nose

     c)   mouth   d)   eye socket   _____

12. The mandible, or lower jawbone, is the:

     a)   largest bone of the face   b)   thinnest bone of the face

     c)   weakest bone of the face   d)   smallest bone of the face   _____

13. The supraorbital nerve is a branch of the:

     a)   mental nerve   b)   auriculotemporal nerve

     c)   fifth cranial nerve   d)   cervical nerve   _____

14. The zygomatic bones form the:

     a)   prominence of the cheeks   b)   sides and crown of the cranium

     c)   upper jaw   d)   bridge of the nose   _____

15. The nasal bones form the:

     a)   forehead   b)   outer ears

     c)   bridge of the nose   d)   tip of the nose   _____

16. The ulnar and radial arteries are the main blood supply of the:

     a)   back of the head   b)   arms and hands

     c)   muscles of the eye   d)   forehead   _____

17. The epicranius muscle covers the:

     a)   side of the head   b)   back of the neck

     c)   bridge of the nose   d)   top of the skull   _____

18. The radial nerve supplies the:

     a)   thumb side of the arm   b)   little finger side of the arm

     c)   palm of the hand   d)   fingers   _____

19. The respiratory system uses spongy tissues in the breathing cycle called the:

     a)   lungs   b)   inhalation

     c)   diaphragm   d)   kidneys   _____

20. Epithelial tissue performs the function of:

     a)   covering body surfaces   b)   contracting and moving parts of the body

     c)   carrying messages to and from the brain   d)   binding together other tissues   _____

21. The circulatory system controls the circulation of blood through the body by means of the heart and:

     a)   pericardium   b)   cervical nerves

     c)   atrium   d)   blood vessels   _____

22. Platelets, which contribute to the blood-clotting process, are also called:

    a) capillaries
    b) leukocytes
    c) erythrocytes
    d) thrombocytes

    _____

23. The internal carotid artery is part of the:

    a) radial arteries
    b) veins of the head, face, and neck
    c) Lymphatics
    d) common carotid artery

    _____

24. Veins are thin-walled vessels that carry blood containing waste products to the heart from the:

    a) capillaries
    b) leukocytes
    c) arteries
    d) lymph nodes

    _____

25. Red blood cells contain hemoglobin and are also called red corpuscles or:

    a) erythrocytes
    b) white blood cells
    c) thrombocytes
    d) plasma

    _____

26. The cervical cutaneous nerve is one of the cervical nerves affecting the:

    a) front and sides of the neck
    b) parotid gland
    c) scalp and muscles behind the ear
    d) scalp at the top of the head

    _____

27. The skeletal system is important because it:

    a) supplies the body with blood
    b) covers and shapes the skeleton
    c) controls and coordinates all other systems
    d) is the physical foundation of the body

    _____

28. Osteology is the scientific study of the:

    a) muscles
    b) nerves
    c) hair
    d) bones

    _____

29. A collection of similar cells that perform a particular function is called a/an:

    a) gland
    b) tissue
    c) organ
    d) system

    _____

30. Protoplasm is the substance that makes up:

    a) all liquid substances
    b) body structures visible to the naked eye
    c) microscopic body structures
    d) the cells of all living things

    _____

31. Blood appears bright red in the arteries (except for the pulmonary artery) and dark red in the:

    a) lymph
    b) corpuscles
    c) aorta
    d) veins

    _____

32. The cranium is the part of the skull that:

   a)   forms the upper jaw
   b)   forms the lower jawbone
   c)   protects the brain
   d)   forms the forehead

   _____

33. Anatomy is the branch of science that studies the:

   a)   minute structures of organic tissues
   b)   functions and activities performed by body structures
   c)   nature, structure, function, and diseases of the muscles
   d)   structures of the human body visible to the naked eye

   _____

34. The middle temporal artery supplies blood to the:

   a)   chin and lower lip
   b)   arms and hands
   c)   side and crown of the head
   d)   temples

   _____

35. The ulna and the radius are the two bones in the:

   a)   wrist
   b)   neck
   c)   upper arm
   d)   forearm

   _____

36. The arteries are thick-walled vessels that carry oxygenated blood away from the heart to the:

   a)   veins
   b)   capillaries
   c)   lymph nodes
   d)   leukocytes

   _____

37. The buccal nerve affects the muscles of the:

   a)   eyebrow
   b)   chin
   c)   side of the neck
   d)   mouth

   _____

38. The atria are the upper, thin-walled chambers of the:

   a)   ventricle
   b)   artery
   c)   pericardium
   d)   heart

   _____

39. Anabolism is the phase of metabolism in which:

   a)   cells divide into two new cells
   b)   complex compounds are broken down into smaller ones
   c)   blood is circulated through the body
   d)   larger molecules are built from smaller ones

   _____

40. The cell membrane is the structure that encloses:

   a)   the nucleus
   b)   living plant and animal cells
   c)   proteins
   d)   the heart

   _____

41. The axon is the part of the nerve cell, or neuron, that:

   a)   both sends and receives impulses
   b)   sends impulses from the cell body
   c)   is within the cell body
   d)   receives impulses from other neurons

   _____

42. Hormones are secreted into:

   a)   the bloodstream   b)   exocrine glands
   c)   the digestive system   d)   ducts   _____

43. Lymph is a clear yellowish fluid that circulates in the:

   a)   lymph vascular system   b)   blood vascular system
   c)   corpuscles   d)   valves   _____

44. The brain is the body's:

   a)   smallest nerve tissue   b)   simplest muscle tissue
   c)   most complex nerve tissue   d)   most complex muscle tissue   _____

45. The superior labial artery is one of the branches of the:

   a)   internal carotid artery   b)   ulnar artery
   c)   angular artery   d)   external maxillary artery   _____

46. The nasal nerve affects the:

   a)   skin of the lower eyelid   b)   skin of the chin
   c)   skin above the temple   d)   point and lower side of the nose   _____

47. One of the critical functions blood performs is:

   a)   carrying carbon dioxide to all body cells   b)   protecting the body from harmful bacteria
   c)   varying the body's temperature   d)   manufacturing toxins   _____

48. The fifth cranial nerve, also called the trifacial or trigeminal nerve, serves as the motor nerve of the muscles that:

   a)   control chewing   b)   affect the eyebrow
   c)   affect the skin between the eyes   d)   control facial expressions   _____

49. The capillaries are blood vessels that connect the smaller arteries to the:

   a)   plasma   b)   valves
   c)   veins   d)   lymph nodes   _____

50. The production of red and white blood cells is one of the functions of the:

   a)   bones   b)   heart
   c)   glands   d)   muscles   _____